Drug calculations for nurses

a step by step approach

Robert Lapham
Pharmacy, St George's Hospital, London, UK
and

Heather Agar
Staff Nurse, Trauma and Orthopaedics,
Charing Cross Hospital, London, UK

ARNOLD

A member of the Hodder Headline Group
LONDON • SYDNEY • AUCKLAND

First published in Great Britain 1995 by
Arnold, a division of Hodder Headline PLC,
338 Euston Road, London NWI 3BH

Whilst the advice and information in this book is believed to be true and
accurate at the date of going to press, neither the authors nor the publisher
can accept any legal responsibility or liability for any errors or omissions
that may be made. In particular (but without limiting the generality of the
preceding disclaimer) every effort has been made to check drug dosages;
however, it is still possible that errors have been missed. Furthermore,
dosage schedules are constantly being revised and new side-effects
recognized. For these reasons the reader is strongly urged to consult the
drug companies' printed instructions before administering any of the drugs
recommended in this book.

British Library Cataloguing in Publication Data
A catalogue record for this book is available from the British Library

Library of Congress Cataloging-in-Publication Data
A catalog record for this book is available from the Library of Congress

ISBN 0 340 604794 (pb)

1 2 3 4 5 95 96 97 98 99

Typeset in 10/12 pt Times by Colset Pte Ltd, Singapore
Printed and bound by JW Arrowsmith Ltd, Bristol.

Contents

Preface
....

Drug treatments given to patients in hospital are becoming increasingly complex. Sometimes, these treatment regimens involve potent and, at times, novel drugs. Many of these drugs are toxic or possibly fatal if administered incorrectly or in overdose. Therefore, it is very important to be able to carry out drug calculations correctly so as not to put the patient at risk.

In current nursing practice, the need to calculate drug dosages is not uncommon. These calculations have to be performed competently and accurately, not only so as not to put the nurse at risk but, more importantly, not to put the patient at risk. This book aims to provide an aid to the basics of mathematics and drug calculations. It is intended to be of use to all nurses of all grades and specialities, and to be a handy reference on the ward.

The idea for this book came from nurses themselves. A frequently asked question was: 'Can you help me with drug calculations?'. Initially, a small booklet was written to help nurses with their drug calculations, particularly those studying for their I.V. certificate. This was very well received, and a questionnaire was sent to nurses asking them what they would like to see featured in a more comprehensive book on drug calculations. As a result, this book was written.

Although this book is primarily for nurses, it may also be helpful to others who use drug calculations in their work. Some subjects have been dealt with in greater detail for this reason, e.g. moles and millimoles. The book should be useful to anyone who wishes to improve their skills in drug calculations or as a refresher course.

Robert Lapham
Heather Agar
1995

How to Use This Book
....

This book is designed for self-study.

Start with the pre-test to assess your current ability in carrying out drug calculations. After completing the book, or relevant sections, the pre-test should be repeated and the two scores compared to see if any improvement has been made.

To attain maximum benefit from the book, start at the beginning and work through one section at a time. For each section attempted, you should fully understand it and be able to answer the problems confidently before moving on to the next section.

Remember

If you are in any doubt about a calculation you are asked to do on the ward – STOP and get help!

1 Pre-test

To obtain the maximum benefit from this book, it is a good idea to attempt the pre-test before you start in order to assess your ability at drug calculations.

The pre-test is divided into several sections which correspond to the sections in the book, and the questions reflect the topics covered by each section. You don't have to attempt every section, only the ones that you feel are relevant to you. Answering the questions will help you identify particular calculations you have difficulty with.

You can use calculators or anything else you find helpful to answer the questions, but it is best to complete the pre-test on your own, as it is *your* ability that is being assessed and not someone else's. Don't worry if you can't answer all of the questions, the aim is to help you to identify areas of weakness.

Once you have completed the pre-test and checked you answers, you can start using the book. Concentrate particularly on the sections you were weak on and, if necessary, miss out the sections you were confident with.

QUESTIONS

Section 2: Basics

The aim of this section is to test your ability on basic principles such as fractions, decimals, powers and using calculators before you start any drug calculations.

Fractions
Solve the following, leaving your answer as a fraction:

1. $\dfrac{5}{9} \times \dfrac{3}{7}$

2. $\dfrac{3}{4} \div \dfrac{9}{16}$

Convert the following to a decimal:

3. $\dfrac{2}{5}$

Decimals
Solve the following:

4. 0.25×0.45

5. $3.5 \div 0.2$

6. 1.38×100

7. $25.64 \div 1,000$

Convert the following to a fraction:

8. 1.2

Powers
Convert the following to a proper number:

9. 3×10^5

Convert the following number to a power of 10:

10. $5,000,000$

Section 3: Units and equivalences

This section is designed to test your knowledge on units normally used in clinical medicine, and how to convert from one unit to another. It is important that you can convert units easily, as this is the basis for most drug calculations.

Convert the following:

Units of weight

1. 0.0625 milligrams   _____ micrograms

2. 600 grams   _____ kilograms

3. 50 nanograms   _____ micrograms

Units of volume

4. 0.15 litres   _____ millilitres

Units of amount of substance

Usually describes the amount of electrolytes, as in an infusion (see Section 8 on Moles and millimoles for a full explanation).

5. 0.36 moles   _____ millimoles

Section 4: Dosage calculations

These are the type of calculations you will be doing every day on the ward.

Drug dosage

Sometimes the dose is given on a body weight basis or in terms of body surface area. The following tests your ability at calculating doses:

1. Dose = 3 mcg/kg/min   Weight = 73 kg
   Dose required = _____ mcg/min
2. Dose = 1.5 mg/m^2 Surface area = 1.55 m^2
   Dose required = _____ mg

Calculating dosages

Calculate how much you need for the following dosages:

3. You have aminophylline injection 250 mg in 10 ml; amount required = 350 mg.
4. You have digoxin injection 500 mcg/2 ml; amount required = 0.75 mg.
5. You have morphine sulphate elixir 10 mg in 5 ml; amount required = 15 mg.

6. You have disopyramide injection 10 mg/1 ml, 5 ml ampoules. Amount required = 300 mg; how many ampoules?

Section 5: Percent and percentages

This section is designed to see if you understand the concept of percent and percentages.

1. How much is 28% of 250 g?
2. What percentage is 160 g of 400 g?

Section 6: Drug strengths or concentrations

This section is designed to see if you understand the various ways in which drug strengths can be expressed.

Percentage concentration

1. How much sodium (in grams) is there in a 500 ml infusion of sodium chloride 1.8%?
2. You need to add 2 g of potassium chloride to a litre of sodium chloride 0.9% infusion. You have 10 ml ampoules of 20% potassium chloride. What volume of potassium chloride do you need to draw up?

mg/ml concentrations

3. What is the concentration (in mg/ml) of an 8.4% sodium bicarbonate infusion?
4. You need to give a 50 mg dose of oral morphine sulphate to a patient. You have a bottle of morphine sulphate elixir at concentration of 2 mg/ml. How much do you need to give for your dose?

'1 in . . .' concentrations or ratio strengths

5. You have a 10 ml ampoule of adrenaline 1 in 10,000. How much adrenaline (in milligrams) does the ampoule contain?

Drugs expressed in units

6. You need to give an infusion of heparin containing 29,000 units over 24 hours. You have ampoules of heparin containing 25,000 units/ml and 5,000 units/ml. How much of each ampoule do you need to draw up?

Section 7: Preparation of solutions (dilutions)

This section is designed to see if you know how to do simple dilutions when making solutions of varying strengths and how to prepare solutions for soaks.

1. You are asked to prepare 3 litres of a 60% solution. How much of your stock solution do you need which diluted to 3 litres will give a 60% solution?
2. You are asked to prepare 5 litres of a 1 in 4,000 solution of potassium permanganate for a soak. You have a solution of potassium permanganate 10 g/litre. How much of your stock solution do you need to dilute to make 5 litres of your soak?

Section 8: Moles and millimoles

This section is designed to see if you understand the concept of millimoles. Millimoles are used to describe the 'amount of substance', and are usually the units for body electrolytes (e.g. sodium 138 mmol/L).

The following questions test your knowledge of various millimole calculations.

Note that the molecular weight of sodium chloride is 58.5.

1. Approximately how many millimoles of sodium are there in a 10 ml ampoule of sodium chloride 30% injection?
2. Approximately how many mmol per litre of sodium are there in an infusion containing 1,800 mg of sodium chloride per litre?

Section 9: Infusion rate calculations

This section tests your knowledge of various infusion rate calculations. It is designed to see if you know the different drop factors for different giving sets and fluids, as well as being able to convert volumes to drops and vice versa.

Calculation of drip rates

1. What is the rate required to give 500 ml of sodium chloride 0.9% infusion over 6 hours using a standard giving set?
2. What is the rate required to give 1 unit of blood (500 ml) over 8 hours using a standard giving set?
3. You are asked to give a 250 ml infusion to a child over 8 hours. What rate should the infusion run using a microdrop (paediatric) giving set?

Conversion of infusion rates (ml/hour) to drops/min
Sometimes, in order to give an infusion, you may need to convert the rate from ml/hour to drops/min.

4. You are asked to give a 1 litre infusion of sodium chloride 0.9% at a rate of 125 ml/hour using a standard giving set. What is the rate in drops/min?

Conversion of dosages to drops/min and ml/hour
Sometimes it may be necessary to convert a dose (mg/min) to an infusion rate (drops/min).

5. You are asked to give 500 ml of doxapram 0.2% infusion at a rate of 3 mg/min using a standard giving set. What is the rate in drops/min? What is the rate in ml/hour?

Conversion of ml/hour to mcg/kg/min or mg/min
With infusion pumps, it may be necessary to convert from ml/hour to mcg/kg/min or mg/min in order to check the rate at which the pump is set.

6. An infusion pump containing 50 mg of sodium nitroprusside in 50 ml, is running at a rate of 13 ml/hour.

The dose wanted is 3 mcg/kg/min and the patient's weight is 72 kg. Is the pump rate correct?

Calculation of length of time of infusions

Sometimes it may be necessary to calculate the number of hours an infusion should run at a specified rate, e.g. to check the drip rates.

7. You have a 250 ml infusion at a rate of 21 drops/min using a standard giving set. Approximately how long will the infusion run?

Section 10: Paediatric dosage calculations

The principles covered by the other sections apply to paediatric calculations. However, doses are usually based on 'mg/kg', so it is important that you can calculate doses on this basis. Other factors to take into account are displacement volumes for antibiotic injections, body surface area nomograms and how to interpret paediatric dosage books. See Section 10 on Paediatric dosage calculations for a fuller explanation.

1. You need to give trimethoprim to a 7-year-old child weighing 23 kg at a dose of 4 mg/kg twice a day. Trimethoprim suspension comes as a 50 mg in 5 ml suspension. How much do you need for each dose?
2. You need to give benzylpenicillin at a dose of 25 mg/kg four times a day to 6-month-old baby weighing 8 kg. How much do you need to draw up for each dose assuming each 600 mg vial is to be reconstituted to 2 ml?

ANSWERS

Section 2: Basics

Fractions

1. $\dfrac{5}{21}$

2. $\dfrac{4}{3}$

3. 0.4

Decimals

4. 0.1125
5. 17.5
6. 138
7. 0.02564

8. $\dfrac{6}{5}$

Powers

9. 300,000
10. 5×10^6

Section 3: Units and equivalences

Units of weight

1. 62.5 micrograms
2. 0.6 kilograms
3. 0.05 micrograms

Units of volume

4. 150 millilitres

Units of amount of substance

5. 360 millimoles

Section 4: Dosage calculations

Drug dosage

1. 219 mcg/min
2. 2.325 mg

Calculating dosages

3. 14 ml
4. 3 ml
5. 7.5 ml
6. 6 ampoules

Section 5: Percent and percentages

1. 70 g
2. 40%

Section 6: Drug strengths or concentrations

Percentage concentration

1. 9 g
2. 10 ml

mg/ml concentrations

3. 84 mg/ml
4. 25 ml

'1 in . . .' concentrations or ratio strengths

5. 1 mg

Drugs expressed in units

6. 1 × 25,000 units/ml ampoule *plus*
  0.8 ml of a 5,000 units/ml ampoule

Section 7: Preparation of solutions (dilutions)

1. 1.8 litres (1,800 ml)
2. 125 ml

Section 8: Moles and millimoles

1. 51.3 mmol (51 mmol)
2. 30.8 mmol (31 mmol)

Section 9: Infusion rate calculations

Calculation of drip rates

1. 27.7 drops/min   (28 drops/min)
2. 15.625 drops/min   (16 drops/min)
3. 31.3 drops/min   (31 drops/min)

Conversion of infusion rates (ml/hour) to drops/min

4. 41.67 drops/min   (42 drops/min)

Conversion of dosages to drops/min and ml/hour

5. 30 drops/min; 90 ml/hour

Conversion of ml/hour to mcg/kg/min or mg/min

6. Dose = 3 mcg/kg/min, so the pump rate is correct.

Calculation of length of time of infusions

7. 238 min = 3 hours 58 min (approx. 4 hours)

Section 10: Paediatric dosage calculations

1. 9 ml
2. 0.67 ml

2 *Basics*

INTRODUCTION

Before dealing with any drug calculations, we will briefly go over a few basic mathematical concepts that may be helpful in some calculations.

This section is designed for those who might want to refresh their memories, particularly those who are returning to nursing after a long absence. If you feel such a refresher course is not necessary, simply miss out this section.

FRACTIONS AND DECIMALS

A basic knowledge of fractions and decimals is helpful since the vast majority of calculations will involve fractions and decimals.

It is important to know how to multiply and divide fractions and decimals, as well as to be able to convert from a fraction to a decimal and vice versa.

Fractions

Before we look at fractions, a few points need to be defined to make explanations easier.

Definition of a fraction

A fraction is part of a whole number or one number divided by another

For example:

$$\frac{2}{5}$$

is a fraction and means 2 parts of 5 (where 5 is the whole).

The number above the 'line' is called the **numerator**. It indicates the number of parts of the whole number that are being used (i.e., in the above example, 2).

The number below the 'line' is called the **denominator**, and it indicates the number of parts into which the whole is divided.

Thus in the example ($\frac{2}{5}$), it means that the whole has been divided into 5 equal parts.

$\frac{2}{5}$ NUMERATOR
DENOMINATOR

Reducing fractions

When you haven't a calculator handy, it is often easier to work with fractions that have been 'simplified' or 'reduced' to their lowest terms.

To reduce a fraction, choose any number which divides exactly into the **numerator** (number on the top) *and* the **denominator** (number on the bottom).

A fraction is said to have been reduced to its lowest terms when it is no longer possible to divide the numerator and denominator by the same number.

Remember
Reducing or simplifying a fraction to its lowest terms does not change the value of the fraction.

EXAMPLES

1. $\dfrac{\overset{3}{\cancel{15}}}{\underset{5}{\cancel{25}}} = \dfrac{3}{5}$ 2. $\dfrac{\overset{\overset{3}{\cancel{27}}}{\cancel{135}}}{\underset{\underset{7}{\cancel{63}}}{\cancel{315}}} = \dfrac{3}{7}$

Remember
− any number that ends in 0 or 5 is divisible by 5
− any even number is divisible by 2
− there can be more than one step (see example 2)

If you have a calculator, then there is no need to reduce fractions to their lowest terms: the calculator does all the hard work for you!

Multiplying fractions
If, at any time, it is necessary to multiply fractions, then it is quite easy to do.

You simply multiply all the numbers 'above the line' (the numerators) and the numbers 'below the line' (the denominators).

For example:

$$\frac{2}{5} \times \frac{3}{7} = \frac{2 \times 3}{5 \times 7} = \frac{6}{35}$$

However, it may be possible to 'simplify' the fraction before multiplying, i.e.

$$\frac{\overset{3}{\cancel{9}}}{\underset{5}{\cancel{15}}} \times \frac{2}{5} = \frac{3 \times 2}{5 \times 5} = \frac{6}{25}$$

In this case, the first fraction has been reduced to its lowest terms by dividing both the numerator and denominator by 3.

You can also 'reduce' both fractions by dividing diagonally by a common number, i.e.

$$\frac{\overset{2}{\cancel{6}}}{7} \times \frac{5}{\underset{3}{\cancel{9}}} = \frac{2 \times 5}{7 \times 3} = \frac{10}{21}$$

In this case, in both fractions there is a number that is divisible by 3 (6 and 9). This is called **cancellation**.

Dividing fractions
Sometimes it may be necessary to divide fractions. You will probably encounter fractions expressed or written like this:

$$\frac{\dfrac{2}{5}}{\dfrac{3}{7}} \quad \text{or} \quad \frac{2}{5} \div \frac{3}{7}$$

In this case, you simply invert the bottom or second fraction and multiply, i.e.

$$\frac{2}{5} \times \frac{7}{3} = \frac{2 \times 7}{5 \times 3} = \frac{14}{15}$$

If, after inverting, reduction or cancellation can occur, then this can be done before multiplying. For example,

$$\frac{5}{2} \div \frac{25}{8}$$

becomes:

$$\frac{\overset{1}{\cancel{5}}}{\underset{1}{\cancel{2}}} \times \frac{\overset{4}{\cancel{8}}}{\underset{5}{\cancel{25}}} = \frac{1 \times 4}{1 \times 5} = \frac{4}{5}$$

Converting fractions to decimals
This is quite easy to do. You simply divide the top number (numerator) by the bottom number (denominator).

If we use our original example:

$$\frac{2}{5} = 2 \div 5$$

$$\begin{array}{r} 0.40 = 0.4 \\ 5\overline{)2.00} \\ \underline{2.0} \\ 0 \end{array}$$

It is important to place the decimal point in the correct position, usually after the number that is being divided (in this case it is 2).

Decimals

Decimals describe 'tenths' of a number, i.e. in terms of 10.

A decimal number consists of a decimal point and numbers both to the left and right of that decimal point. Just as whole numbers have positions for units, tens, hundreds etc., so do decimal numbers, but on *both* sides of the decimal point, i.e.

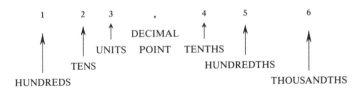

Numbers to the **left** of the decimal point are **greater than one**.
Numbers to the **right** of the decimal point are **less than one**.

Thus

1.25 is equal to **one** plus a **fraction of one**

0.25 is equal to a **fraction of one**

Multiplying decimals

Decimals are multiplied in the same way as whole numbers except there is a decimal point to worry about.

If you don't have a calculator handy, as stated before, it is important to put the decimal point in the correct place in the answer.

Consider the sum

$$0.65 \times 0.75$$

$$
\begin{array}{r}
0.65 \\
\times \ \underline{0.75} \\
325 \\
\underline{4550} \\
4875
\end{array}
$$

You may use another method, but the answer should be the same.

The decimal point is placed as many places to the **left** as there are numbers after it in the sum (i.e. in this case there are four).

$$0 \cdot 6\,5 \times 0 \cdot 7\,5$$

$$\quad 1\;2 \qquad 3\;4 = 4$$

Therefore in the answer, the decimal point is moved four places to the **left**.

$$. \overgroup{4\;8\;7\;5} = 0.4875$$

The following is a quick method for multiplying by multiples of 10.

You simply move the decimal point the number of places to the **right** as there are noughts or zeros in the number you are multiplying by.

For example, if you are multiplying by 10, 100, 1,000 or 10,000, see Table 2.1.

TABLE 2.1 Multiplying decimals

Multiplying by (number)	Number of zeros	Move the decimal point (to the right)
10	1	1 place
100	2	2 places
1,000	3	3 places
10,000	4	4 places etc.

Dividing decimals

Division of decimals is quite simple, but once again the placement of the decimal point is important.

To make it easier to explain, the following terms are used:

$$\frac{\text{DIVIDEND}}{\text{DIVISOR}} = \text{QUOTIENT (answer)} \quad or$$

$$\text{DIVISOR} \overline{)\,\text{DIVIDEND}}^{\text{QUOTIENT (answer)}}$$

Consider

$$\frac{34.8}{4} \quad \text{which can be rewritten as} \quad 4\overline{)34.8}$$

The decimal point in the answer (quotient) is placed directly above the decimal point in the dividend:

```
      8 . 7
4 )34 . 8
   32
   ──
   28
```

However, if you are dividing a decimal by another decimal, then it is slightly different.

Consider

$$\frac{1.55}{0.2} \qquad 0.2\overline{)1.55}$$

Make the **divisor** equal to a **whole number**, i.e. in this case, move the decimal point **one** place to the **right**.

Move the decimal point in the **dividend** the **same number** of places to the **right**.

In this case

$$0\,.\,\overset{\frown}{2} \qquad 1\,.\,\overset{\frown}{5}\,5$$

which equals

$$2\overline{)15.5}$$

Then the decimal point in the answer (**quotient**) is placed directly above the decimal point in the dividend as before.

```
    7 . 75
2 )15 . 5
   14
   ‾‾
   15
   14
   ‾‾
   10
```

It is quite easy if you are dividing by multiples of 10.

You simply move the decimal point the number of places to the **left** as there are noughts or zeros in the number you are dividing by.

For example, if you are dividing by 10, 100, 1,000 or 10,000, see Table 2.2.

TABLE 2.2 Dividing decimals

Dividing by (number)	Number of zeros	Move the decimal point (to the left)
10	1	1 place
100	2	2 places
1,000	3	3 places
10,000	4	4 places etc.

EXAMPLE

$$\frac{546}{100}$$

Move the decimal point **three** place to the **left** (there are three zeros in the bottom number):

0 . 5 4 6

Rounding of decimal numbers

Sometimes it is necessary to 'round up' or 'round down' a decimal number to a whole number.

This is particularly true in infusion rate calculations, as it is impossible to give a part of a drop when setting an infusion rate.

If the number after the decimal point is 4 or less, then ignore it, i.e. 'round down'.

For example:

31.25

The number after the decimal point is 4 or less, so it becomes

31

If the number after the decimal point is 5 or more, then add 1 to the whole number, i.e. 'round up'.

For example:

41.67

The number after the decimal point is 5 or more, so it becomes

42

Converting decimals to fractions

It is unlikely that you would want to convert a decimal to a fraction in any calculation, but this is included here just in case.

First you have to make the decimal a whole number by moving the decimal point to the **right**, i.e.

$0 \,.\, \overgroup{7\ 5}$ becomes 75 (the **numerator** in the fraction)

Next divide by a multiple of 10 (the **denominator**) to make a fraction.

The value of this multiple of 10 is determined by how many places to the **right** the decimal point has moved, i.e.

1 place = a denominator of 10
2 places = a denominator of 100
3 places = a denominator of 1,000

Thus in our example

0.75 = 75 (decimal point has moved 2 places to the right)

Therefore the denominator = 100:

$\dfrac{75}{100} = \dfrac{3}{4}$ (divide the numerator and denominator by 25)

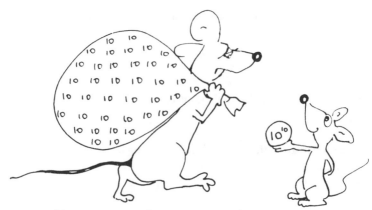

Use a power to make cumbersome
numbers more manageable

POWERS

Powers or exponentials are a convenient way of writing very large or very small numbers. Here, we will briefly look at powers of 10, as it is these you will meet in your calculations.

Consider the following:

$$10 \times 10 \times 10 \times 10 \times 10$$

You are repeatedly multiplying by 10. In short you can write:

10^5 instead of $10 \times 10 \times 10 \times 10 \times 10$

The small raised number 5 next to the 10 is known as the **power** – it tells you how many of the same number are being multiplied together.

$10^5 \longleftarrow$ POWER

It is known as '10 to the power of 5' or just '10 to the 5'.

Now consider this:

$$\frac{1}{10} \times \frac{1}{10} \times \frac{1}{10} \times \frac{1}{10} \times \frac{1}{10} = \frac{1}{10 \times 10 \times 10 \times 10 \times 10}$$

You are repeatedly dividing by 10. In short you can write:

10^{-5} instead of $\dfrac{1}{10 \times 10 \times 10 \times 10 \times 10}$

In this case, you will notice that there is a minus sign next to the power.

$$10^{-5} \longleftarrow \text{MINUS POWER}$$

It is a **negative power**, and is known as '10 to the power of minus 5' or just '10 to the minus 5'.

In conclusion:

A positive power means MULTIPLY by the number of times of the power

A negative power means DIVIDE by the number of times of the power

However, you will probably come across powers used as in the following:

$$3 \times 10^3 \quad \text{or} \quad 5 \times 10^{-2}$$

This is known as the **standard index form**. It is a combination of a power of 10 and a number with one unit in front of a decimal point, i.e.

$$5 \times 10^6 \quad (5.0 \times 10^6)$$
$$1.2 \times 10^3$$
$$4.5 \times 10^{-2}$$
$$3 \times 10^{-6} \quad (3.0 \times 10^{-6})$$

The number in front of the decimal point can be anything from 0 to 9.

This type of notation is the type seen on a calculator when describing very large or small numbers. It is a common and convenient way of describing numbers without having to write a lot of noughts.

Here are some more examples:

$$3 \times 10^5 \quad = 3 \times 100,000$$
$$1.4 \times 10^3 \quad = 1.4 \times 1,000$$
$$4 \times 10^{-2} = 4 \div 100$$
$$2.25 \times 10^{-3} = 2.25 \div 1,000$$

Because you are dealing in tens, you will notice that the 'number of noughts' you multiply or divide by is equal to the power.

Thus

(1) 3×10^5

TABLE 2.3 Powers of 10

Power of 10	Standard form
10^9	1,000,000,000
10^8	100,000,000
10^7	10,000,000
10^6	1,000,000
10^5	100,000
10^4	10,000
10^3	1,000
10^2	100
10^1	10
10^{-1}	0.1
10^{-2}	0.01
10^{-3}	0.001
10^{-4}	0.0001
10^{-5}	0.00001
10^{-6}	0.000001
10^{-7}	0.0000001
10^{-8}	0.00000001
10^{-9}	0.000000001

You move the decimal point **five** places to the **right** (positive power of 5), so it becomes

$$3 \times 10^5 = 3\ 0\ 0\ 0\ 0\ 0\ . = 300,000$$

5 noughts

(2) 4×10^{-2}

You move the decimal point **two** places to the **left** (negative power of 2), so it becomes

$$4 \times 10^{-2} = 0\ .\ 0\ 4 = 0.04$$

2 noughts

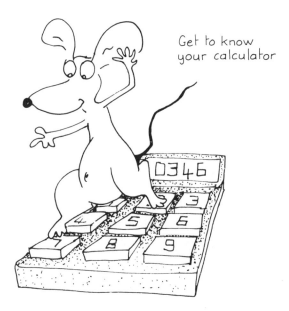

Get to know
your calculator

USE OF CALCULATORS

Always consult the manual or instructions that came with your calculator. Note that numbers should be entered in a certain way when using a calculator and you need to know how to read the display.

This next section will hopefully explain how to use your calculator properly.

Consider the following:

$$\frac{2}{500} \times 140$$

There are two ways of entering this into your calculator:

Method 1:

Enter [2]	DISPLAY = 2
Enter [×]	DISPLAY = 2
Enter [1] [4] [0]	DISPLAY = 140

You are doing the sum: *2 × 140*

Enter [÷]	DISPLAY = 280
Enter [5] [0] [0]	DISPLAY = 500

You are doing the sum: $\dfrac{2 \times 140}{500}$

   Enter [=]   DISPLAY = 0.56 (answer)

Method 2:
   Enter [2]   DISPLAY = 2
   Enter [÷]   DISPLAY = 2
   Enter [5] [0] [0]   DISPLAY = 500

You are doing the sum: $\dfrac{2}{500}$

   Enter [×]   DISPLAY = 4^{-03} or 0.004
This notation is the way your calculator shows small numbers
(see 'Powers').
   Enter [1] [4] [0]   DISPLAY = 140

You are doing the sum: $\dfrac{2}{500} \times 140$

   Enter [=]   DISPLAY = 0.56 (answer)

Now consider the following:

$$\frac{20}{60} \times \frac{1,000}{8}$$

Method 1:
   Enter [2] [0]   DISPLAY = 20
   Enter [÷]   DISPLAY = 20
   Enter [6] [0]   DISPLAY = 60

You are doing the sum: $\dfrac{20}{60}$

   Enter [×]   DISPLAY = 0.3333333
   Enter [1] [0] [0] [0]   DISPLAY = 1000

You are doing the sum: $\dfrac{20}{60} \times 1,000$

Enter [÷]   DISPLAY = 333.33333
Enter [8]   DISPLAY = 8

You are doing the sum: $\dfrac{20}{60} \times \dfrac{1,000}{8}$

Enter [=]   DISPLAY = 41.66667 (answer)

Method 2:

Enter [2] [0]   DISPLAY = 20
Enter [×]   DISPLAY = 20
Enter [1] [0] [0] [0]   DISPLAY = 1000

You are doing the sum: $20 \times 1,000$

Enter [÷]   DISPLAY = 20000
Enter [6] [0]   DISPLAY = 60

You are doing the sum: $\dfrac{20 \times 1,000}{60}$

Enter [÷]   DISPLAY = 333.33333
Enter [8]   DISPLAY = 8

You are doing the sum: $\dfrac{20 \times 1,000}{60 \times 8}$

Enter [=]   DISPLAY = 41.66667 (answer)

Whatever method you use, the answer is the same. However, it may be easier to split the sum into two parts, i.e.

(1) $20 \times 1,000$ and
(2) 60×8

Then divide (1) by (2), i.e.

$$\dfrac{20}{60} \times \dfrac{1,000}{8} = \dfrac{20,000}{480} = 41.66667$$

Now consider a sum written as:

$$\dfrac{6}{4 \times 5}$$

You can *either* simplify the sum, i.e. $\frac{6}{20}$, then divide 6 by 20 (= 0.3), *or* enter the following on your calculator:

Enter [6]	DISPLAY = 6
Enter [÷]	DISPLAY = 6
Enter [4]	DISPLAY = 4

You are doing the sum: $\frac{6}{4} = 1.5$

Enter [÷]	DISPLAY = 1.5
Enter [5]	DISPLAY = 5

You are doing the sum: $\dfrac{\frac{6}{4}}{5}$ i.e. $\dfrac{1.5}{5}$

Enter [=]	DISPLAY = 0.3 (answer)

So, in conclusion, you can use either method, but it may be easier to simplify 'above the line' (the top line) and 'below the line' (the bottom line) before dividing the two.

See the section on 'powers' for an explanation of how a scientific calculator displays very large and small numbers.

Powers and calculators

The display on a normal calculator is usually eight numbers:

$$\boxed{9\,9\,9\,9\,9\,9\,9\,9.}$$

The maximum number that can be displayed in this way is therefore:

99,999,999

The smallest number that can be displayed is therefore:

0.0000001

However, on a scientific calculator, if an answer is either larger or smaller than that which can normally be displayed, then the answer will be shown as a power or exponential of 10, i.e.

$$\boxed{5.^{06}}$$

or

$$3.^{-06}$$

As stated before, this is known as **standard index form**.

$5.^{06} = 5 \times 10^6 = 5 \times 1,000,000 = 5,000,000$

$3.^{-06} = 3 \times 10^{-6} = \dfrac{3}{1,000,000} = 0.000003$

So if the answer is displayed like this (the proper name is an **exponential**) on your calculator, you simply move the decimal point the number of places as indicated by the power and to the left or to the right depending on whether it is a negative or positive power.

$5.^{06} = 5 \times 10^6 = 5 \underbrace{0\ 0\ 0\ 0\ 0\ 0}. = 5,000,000$

6 noughts

$3.^{-06} = 3 \times 10^{-6} = \underbrace{0.0\ 0\ 0\ 0\ 0}\ 3 = 0.000003$

6 noughts

MEASURING LIQUIDS

The proper way to measure large volumes is to use a specific measure. However, it is unlikely that you will find a proper measure on the ward; liquids are usually measured with medicine pots and syringes (especially liquids or medicines to be administered to patients).

All three methods of measuring liquids will be covered here.

(1) Cylindrical and conical measures

These measures are mainly used for liquids that are for oral or external use (ranging from 1 ml to 1,000 ml).

Cylindrical measures are more accurate and are mainly used in chemical laboratories; conical flasks or measures are those that are mainly found in dispensaries.

Each measure must bear the stamp of a Weights and Measures Inspector.

When liquid is poured into a measure, the liquid 'clings' to the

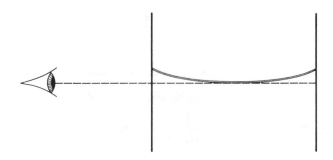

FIGURE 2.1 Meniscus

sides creating a 'curved' level which is known as the **meniscus**. This is due to the surface tension of the liquid.

When measuring, the top of the graduation line must be aligned with the true meniscus, i.e. the lowest part of the liquid (see Figure 2.1).

It is important that the measure should be on a flat surface or held as level as possible. The graduation mark to which you are measuring should be at eye level. If viewed from above, the level may appear higher than it really is; if viewed from below, it appears lower. There are usually guide lines at the back of the measure to help align the meniscus properly, preventing these eye level errors.

For good practice, the most appropriate measure should be chosen. If possible, do not split the volume between two measures because this increases errors, i.e. if measuring 300 ml, a 500 ml measure would be better than measuring 100 ml and 200 ml.

When pouring, carefully pour the liquid into the centre of the measure; any that falls on to the sides above the relevant graduation mark has to be allowed to drain down before adjusting to the final volume.

(2) Measuring pots
These are used on the ward to measure individual patient doses. They measure volumes ranging from 5 ml to 30 ml, and are not meant to be accurate. However, the same principles apply when using measuring pots: measure at eye level.

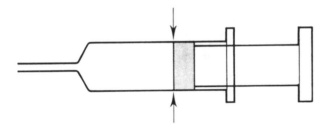

FIGURE 2.2

(3) Syringes

When measuring volumes with syringes, it is important to expel all the air first before adjusting to the final volume. The volume is measured from the bottom of the plunger (Figure 2.2).

The small amount of liquid that is left in the nozzle of the syringe after administering the drug is already taken into account by the manufacturer when calibrating the syringe. Therefore you shouldn't try and administer this small volume: this is known as 'dead space' or 'dead volume' (Figure 2.3).

Once again, you should use the most appropriate syringe for your dose.

It is important that injection doses are measured correctly: an overdose can be dangerous; too low a dose may result in an ineffective dose.

When calculating doses for injections, the number of decimal places in the answer should match the graduations on the syringe being used (see Table 2.4).

For example, if you are going to use a 2 ml syringe with 0.1 ml graduations, you would calculate and 'round up' your answer to

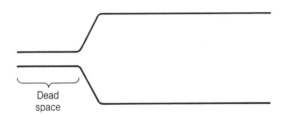

Dead
space

FIGURE 2.3

one decimal place, i.e.

1. Your answer = 1.63 ml, you would draw up 1.6 ml
2. Your answer = 1.68 ml, you would draw up 1.7 ml

Examples are given in Table 2.5.

TABLE 2.4 Syringe calibrations

1 ml syringe = 0.1 ml	divisions subdivided into 0.01 ml	graduations
2 ml syringe = 0.5 ml	divisions subdivided into 0.1 ml	graduations
5 ml syringe = 1 ml	divisions subdivided into 0.5 ml	graduations
10 ml syringe = 1 ml	divisions subdivided into 0.5 ml	graduations
20 ml syringe = 5 ml	divisions subdivided into 1 ml	graduations
50 ml syringe = 10 ml	divisions subdivided into 1 ml	graduations

TABLE 2.5 Accuracy of syringe calculations

1 ml syringe, 0.01 ml	graduations, answers to **two** decimal places
2 ml syringe, 0.1 ml	graduations, answers to **one** decimal place
5 ml syringe, 0.5 ml	graduations, answers to **one** decimal place
10 ml syringe, 0.5 ml	graduations, answers to **one** decimal place

3 Units and equivalences

....

OBJECTIVES

At the end of this section, you should be familiar with the following:

Basic units

Prefixes used in clinical medicine

Equivalences

Equivalences of weight

Equivalences of volume

Equivalences of amount of substance

Conversion from one unit to another

INTRODUCTION

There are many different units used in medicine. For example:

Drug strengths:	digoxin injection 500 mcg in 1 ml
Dosages:	dobutamine 3 mcg/kg/min
Patient electrolyte levels:	sodium 137 mmol/L

and many more.

Therefore it is important to have a basic knowledge of the units used in medicine and how they are derived.

It is particularly important to have an understanding of the units in which drugs can be prescribed; and how to convert from one unit to another – this last part is very important as it is the basis of all drug calculations.

UNITS

The International System of Units (S.I.) or metric system has been generally accepted in the United Kingdom and certain other countries for use in medical practice and pharmacy.

The main units are those of:

> Weight
> Volume
> Amount of substance

TABLE 3.1 S.I. base units

Quantity	Name of unit	Unit symbol
Weight	Kilogram	kg
Volume	Litre	L or l
Amount of substance	Mole	mol

TABLE 3.2 Prefixes used in clinical practice

Prefix	Symbol	Division/multiple	Factor
mega	M	×1,000,000	10^6
kilo	k	×1,000	10^3
deci	d	÷10	10^{-1}
centi	c	÷100	10^{-2}
milli	m	÷1,000	10^{-3}
micro	mc	÷1,000,000	10^{-6}
nano	n	÷1,000,000,000	10^{-9}

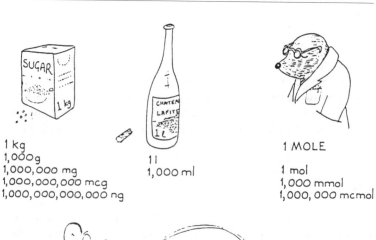

1 kg
1,000 g
1,000,000 mg
1,000,000,000 mcg
1,000,000,000,000 ng

1 l
1,000 ml

1 MOLE

1 mol
1,000 mmol
1,000,000 mcmol

S.I. prefixes

When the S.I. unit is inconveniently large or small, prefixes are used to denote multiples or sub-multiples. In practice, it is preferable to use multiples of a thousand, e.g. gram, milligram, microgram, nanogram.

The main prefixes you will come across on the ward will be:

mega = a unit expressed in terms of millions
milli = a thousandth of a unit
micro = a millionth of a unit
nano = a thousand-millionth of a unit

Thus in practice, drug strengths and dosages can be expressed in various ways, i.e.

1. Benzylpenicillin – sometimes expressed in terms of mega units (1 mega unit means 1 million units of activity). Each vial contains benzylpenicillin 600 mg which equals 1 mega unit.

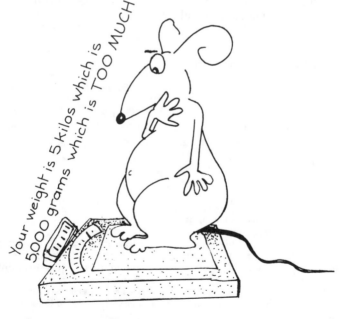

(Equivalents of weight)

2. Liquids are often expressed in millilitres (ml) which are used to describe small volumes, e.g. lactulose, 10 ml to be given three times a day.
3. Drug strengths are usually expressed in milligrams (mg), e.g. frusemide 40 mg tablets.
4. When the amount of drug present is very small, strengths are expressed as either micrograms (mcg) or even nanograms (ng), e.g. digoxin 125 mcg tablets, alfacalcidol 250 ng capsules.

N.B. For the purposes of writing prescriptions the word 'micrograms' should be written in full; when an abbreviation is necessary, the British Pharmacopoeia recommends that 'mcg' be used rather than 'μg'.

EQUIVALENCES

As already stated, S.I. units are too large for everyday clinical use, so they are subdivided into multiples of 1,000.

TABLE 3.3 Equivalences of weight

Unit	Symbol		Equivalent	Symbol
1 kilogram	kg	=	1,000 grams	g
1 gram	g	=	1,000 milligrams	mg
1 milligram	mg	=	1,000 micrograms	mcg
1 microgram	mcg	=	1,000 nanograms	ng

TABLE 3.4 Equivalences of volume

Unit	Symbol	Equivalent	Symbol
1 litre	L or l*	1,000 millilitres	ml

* The official symbol for litres is a small 'L' (l), but this is sometimes mistaken for a 'one' (1), e.g. 2l means 2 litres and not '21'. So sometimes a large 'L' is used to avoid confusion, especially when typed or printed.

TABLE 3.5 Equivalences of amount of substance

Unit	Symbol	Equivalent	Symbol
1 mole	mol	1,000 millimoles	mmol
1 millimole	mmol	1,000 micromoles	mcmol

Moles and millimoles are the terms used by chemists when measuring quantities of certain substances or chemicals; they are more accurate than using grams. For a fuller explanation, see Section 8 on Moles and millimoles.

Examples include:

    0.5 kg   = 500 g
    0.25 g   = 250 mg
    0.2 mg   = 200 mcg
    0.5 L   = 500 ml
    0.25 mol = 250 mmol

CONVERSION FROM ONE UNIT TO ANOTHER

In drug calculations, it is best to work in whole numbers, i. e. 125 mcg and not 0.125 mg, as fewer mistakes are then made. It is always best to work with the smaller unit to avoid decimals and decimal points. Therefore, it is necessary to be able to convert easily from one unit to another. To do this you have to multiply or divide by 1,000.

In general:

To convert from a **larger** unit to a **smaller** unit, **multiply** by 1,000
To convert from a **smaller** unit to a **larger** unit, **divide** by 1,000

In each case, the decimal point moves three places either to the right or to the left, depending upon whether you are converting from a larger unit to a smaller unit or vice versa (see the Worked Examples).

It is important to note that, when converting from a very large unit to a much smaller unit (or vice versa), the conversion may involve two steps.

For example, you wish to convert from kilograms to milligrams. Thus to convert 0.005 kg to milligrams, first convert to grams:

0.005 kg = 0.005 × 1,000 = 5 g

Next, convert grams to milligrams:

5 g = 5 × 1,000 = 5,000 mg

Therefore, it is important to look at the units carefully; converting from one unit to another may involve two steps.

Remember
When converting, the amount remains the same, only the unit changes. Obviously, it appears more when expressed as a smaller unit, but the amount remains the same.

WORKED EXAMPLES

1. Convert 0.5 g to mg.
You are going from a larger unit to a smaller unit. Therefore you have to multiply by 1,000, i.e.

0.5 g × 1,000 = 500 mg

Decimal point moves three places to the right:

0 . 5 0 0 = 500

2. Convert 2,000 g to kg.
You are going from a smaller unit to a larger unit. Therefore you have to divide by 1,000, i.e.

$$2,000 \text{ g} = \frac{2,000}{1,000} = 2 \text{ kg}$$

Decimal point moves three places to the left:

2 0 0 0 . = 2

3. Convert 1.45 L to ml.
You are going from a larger unit to a smaller unit. Therefore you have to multiply by 1,000, i.e.

1.45 L × 1,000 = 1,450 ml

Decimal point moves three places to the right:

$$1 . \overset{\frown}{4} \overset{\frown}{5} \overset{\frown}{0} = 1{,}450$$

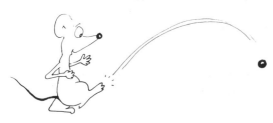

0.125 mg   =   125.0 mcg

To change a larger unit, eg mg, to a smaller unit, eg mcg, <u>multiply</u> by 1000 (ie move the point 3 places to the <u>right</u>)

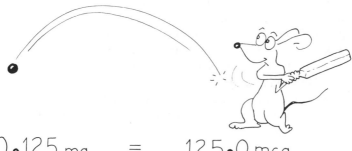

0.125 mg   =   125.0 mcg

To change a smaller unit (eg mcg) to a larger unit (eg mg), divide by 1000 (ie move the point 3 places to the <u>left</u>)

UNITS AND EQUIVALENCES – SUMMARY

To convert a larger unit to a smaller unit – multiply by 1,000

i.e. the decimal point moves three places to the right:

$$0.125 \, \text{mg} = 0 . \overset{\frown}{1} \overset{\frown}{2} \overset{\frown}{5} = 125 \, \text{mcg}$$

To convert from a smaller unit to a larger unit – divide by 1,000

i.e. the decimal point moves three places to the left:

$$125 \, mcg = 0 \, . \, \overbrace{1 \ 2 \ 5} = 0.125 \, mg$$

Remember
Look at the units carefully; converting from one unit to another may involve two steps.

PROBLEMS

A.1 Convert 0.0125 kilograms to grams
A.2 Convert 250 nanograms to micrograms
A.3 Convert 3.2 litres to millilitres
A.4 Convert 0.0273 moles to millimoles
A.5 Convert 3,750 grams to kilograms
A.6 Convert 0.05 grams to micrograms
A.7 Convert 4.5×10^{-6} grams to nanograms
A.8 Convert 25,000 milligrams to kilograms
A.9 You have an ampoule of digoxin 0.5 mg in 2 ml.
How many mcg/ml?
A.10 You have an ampoule of fentanyl 0.05 mg/ml.
How much (in mcg/ml) is there in a 2 ml ampoule?

ANSWERS TO PROBLEMS

A.1 12.5 grams
A.2 0.25 micrograms
A.3 3,200 millilitres
A.4 27.3 millimoles
A.5 3.75 kilograms
A.6 50,000 micrograms
A.7 4,500 nanograms
A.8 0.025 kilograms
A.9 Convert milligrams to micrograms. You are going from a larger unit to a smaller unit, therefore multiply by 1,000:

$$0.5 \, \text{mg} \times 1,000 = 500 \, \text{mcg}$$

Thus you have 500 mcg in 2 ml. Divide by 2 to find out how much is in 1 ml, i.e.

$$\frac{500}{2} = 250 \, \text{mcg}$$

Answer: 250 mcg/ml.

A.10 Convert milligrams to micrograms. You are going from a larger unit to a smaller unit, therefore multiply by 1,000:

$$0.05 \, \text{mg} \times 1,000 = 50 \, \text{mcg}$$

Thus you have 50 mcg in 1 ml. Therefore to find out how much is in a 2 ml ampoule, multiply by 2:

$$50 \, \text{mcg} \times 2 = 100 \, \text{mcg}$$

Answer: 100 mcg in a 2 ml ampoule.

4 *Dosage calculations*
....

OBJECTIVES

At the end of this section, you should be familiar with the following:

Calculate dosages (from body weight or body surface area)

Calculate divided doses

Calculate how much to administer using the 'one unit' rule

Know whether your answer seems reasonable

INTRODUCTION

These are the basic everyday type of calculations you will be doing on the ward.

They include: simple drug dosages; calculating divided doses; and calculating how much you need to give to a patient.

It is important that you are able to do these calculations confidently, as mistakes could result in the patient receiving the wrong dose, with serious consequences.

After completing this section, not only should you be able to do the calculations, but also to decide whether your answer is reasonable.

DRUG DOSAGE

Sometimes, the dose required is calculated on a body weight basis (mg/kg) or in terms of a patient's surface area (mg/m^2) – this particularly applies to cytotoxics and other drugs that require an accurate individual dose.

Thus the dose required for a particular patient depends upon their individual weight or body surface area. (Surface area is calculated from **nomograms** – using patient's height and weight.) Examples of these nomograms, and how to use them, can be found in Appendix 1.

EXAMPLES

1. The dose required is 3 mg/kg and the patient weighs 68 kg.

   This means that for every kilogram (kg) of a patient's weight, you will need 3 mg of drug.

   In this example, the patient weighs 68 kg. Therefore this patient will need 68 lots of 3 mg of drug, i.e. you simply multiply the dose by the patient's weight:

   $3 \, mg/kg = 3 \times 68 = 204 \, mg$

   Thus the patient will need a total dose of 204 mg.

   This can be summarized as:

   Total dose required = Dose/kg × Patient's weight

2. If the dose is given in mg/m^2, you do exactly the same – multiply the dose by the patient's surface area.

   Total dose required = Dose/m² × Body surface area

   The dose required is 500 mg/m^2 and the patient's body surface area equals 1.89 m^2.

   This means that for every square metre (m^2) of a patient's surface area, you will need 500 mg of drug.

   In this example, the patient's body surface area is 1.89 m^2. Therefore this patient will need 1.89 lots of 500 mg of drug, i.e. you simply multiply the dose by the patient's body surface area:

   $500 \, mg/m^2 = 500 \times 1.89 = 945 \, mg$

   Thus the patient will need a total dose of 945 mg.

To find the body surface area for a patient, you will need that patient's weight and height. Then using special tables or nomograms, the body surface area can be calculated.

PROBLEMS

Work out the following dosages:

B.1 Dose = 1.5 mg/kg, patient's weight = 73 kg
B.2 Dose = 8 mg/kg, patient's weight = 64.5 kg
B.3 Dose = 60 mg/kg, patient's weight = 12 kg
B.4 Dose = 0.4 ml/kg, patient's weight = 62 kg
B.5 Dose = 50 mg/m^2, patient's surface area = 1.94 m^2
B.6 Dose = 120 mg/m^2, patient's surface area = 1.55 m^2
B.7 Dose = 400 mcg/kg, patient's weight = 54 kg
  (i) What is the total dose in mcg?
 (ii) What is the total dose in mg?
B.8 Dose = 5 mcg/kg/min, patient's weight = 65 kg
What is the dose in mcg/min?
(You will meet this type of calculation with I.V. infusions – see Section 9.)
B.9 Dose = 3 mcg/kg/min, patient's weight = 85 kg
What is the dose in mcg/min?
B.10 Dose = 500 mcg/kg/min, patient's weight = 78 kg
What is the dose in mg/min?

DIVIDED DOSES

Sometimes the dose of a drug is given as a total daily dose (T.D.D.) which has to be given in divided doses (usually three or four times a day).

It is important that you can tell the difference between the total daily dose (T.D.D.) and individual doses. If not interpreted properly, then the patient is at risk of receiving the T.D.D. as an individual dose, thus receiving three or four times the normal dose (with disastrous results!). This can be a problem with paediatric doses as a lot of the doses are given in reference books as total daily doses (see Section 10 Paediatric dosage calculations).

To illustrate this point, consider the following:

Ibuprofen 1,200 mg daily given three times a day

This is *not* 1,200 mg to be given three times a day, *but* 1,200 mg in three divided doses, i.e.

$$\frac{1,200}{3} = 400 \text{ mg three times a day}$$

The patient is at risk of receiving three times the dose.

Therefore it is very important that doses are read and interpreted properly. **Read the wording carefully**.

With divided doses, simply divide the total daily dose by the number of divided doses.

EXAMPLE

Cefuroxime I.V. 2.25 g in divided doses every 8 hours

Eight-hourly is equal to 3 divided doses (6-hourly would be equal to 4 divided doses). Therefore divide the total daily dose by 3.

In this case, it would be better to convert 2.25 g to milligrams as each dose will have to be given in milligrams:

$$2.25 \text{ g} = 2.25 \times 1,000 = 2,250 \text{ mg}$$

Then divide by 3 to find the amount needed for each dose:

$$\frac{2,250}{3} = 750 \text{ mg}$$

You will need to give cefuroxime I.V. 750 mg every 8 hours (three times a day).

Sometimes it may be necessary to calculate hourly volumes for infusions. In this case simply divide the total volume by the number of hours over which the infusion is to be given.

EXAMPLE

500 ml sodium chloride 0.9% infusion over 8 hours

To find the hourly volume, divide 500 by 8:

$$\frac{500}{8} = 62.5\,ml$$

Knowing the hourly volume is very useful in I.V. calculations. It is used in the formula to calculate infusion drip rates (see Section 9 on Intravenous therapy).

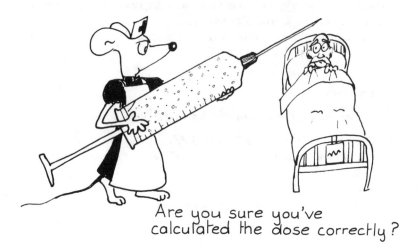

Are you sure you've calculated the dose correctly?

CALCULATING DRUG DOSAGES

There are several ways of solving this type of calculation; it is best to learn one way and stick to it.

The easiest way is by proportion, what you do to one side of an equation, do to the other side.

Whatever the type of calculation you are doing, it is always best to make what you've got equal to **one** and then multiply by what you want. This can be called the '**one** unit' rule. This may sound a bit confusing, but it should appear clearer after working through the worked example.

Also, when what you've got and what you want are in different units, you need to convert everything to the same units. In doing this, it is best to convert to whole numbers to avoid decimal points as fewer mistakes are then made. If possible, it is a good idea to convert everything to the units of the answer.

WORKED EXAMPLE

You need to prepare an infusion of digoxin containing 0.75 mg. Digoxin comes as 500 mcg/2ml. How many ml do you need?

Step 1

The units of what you've got (500 mcg/2 ml) and what you want (0.75 mg) are different. Therefore convert everything to micrograms (mcg), as long as it avoids decimal points.

$$0.75 \, mg = 0.75 \times 1,000 = 750 \, mcg$$

Step 2

Calculate how much **one** unit is of what you have, i.e.

$$500 \, mcg \, in \, 2 \, ml$$

$$1 \, mcg = \frac{2}{500} \, ml$$

This is known as the '**one** unit' rule.

Step 3

But you want to know how much for 750 mcg, therefore multiply the amount from Step 2 by 750.

$$750 \, mcg = \frac{2}{500} \times 750 = 3 \, ml$$

Answer: You will need to draw up 3 ml of digoxin.

A simple formula can be used to calculate drug dosages:

$$\frac{\textbf{Amount you want}}{\textbf{Amount you've got}} \times \textbf{Volume it's in}$$

Once again, in the above Worked Example, before entering numbers in the formula, convert everything to the same units. Thus:

Amount you want   =   750 mcg
Amount you've got   =   500 mcg
Volume it's in   =   2 ml

Substitute the numbers in the formula:

$$\frac{750}{500} \times 2 = 3 \text{ ml}$$

We obtain the same answer, that you will need to draw up 3 ml of digoxin.

You can apply this method to whatever type of calculation you want (not just micrograms and milligrams).

EXAMPLE

You need to add 20 millimoles (mmol) of potassium chloride to an infusion. You have 27 mmol in 10 ml. Therefore

$$1 \text{ mmol} = \frac{10}{27} \text{ ml}$$

Thus for 20 mmol, you will need:

$$\frac{10}{27} \times 20 = 7.4 \text{ ml}$$

It can equally be applied to units as with heparin, and whatever units the drug may be prescribed in.

CHECKING YOUR ANSWER – DOES IT APPEAR REASONABLE?

When doing this sort of calculation, it is good practice to have a rough idea of the answer first, so you can check your final calculated answer.

To illustrate this point, consider the earlier Worked Example: you had digoxin 500 mcg in 2 ml, and you wanted digoxin 750 mcg.

Obviously, the final volume you want will be more than 2 ml but less than 4 ml (4 ml = 1,000 mcg). So the answer will be between 2 and 4 ml. If the answer you get is outside this range, then your answer is wrong and you should re-check your calculations.

As you can see, having a rough idea of the answer before you do your calculation means that you can decide whether the answer you get is reasonable.

Sometimes, it may not be possible to guess your answer (as with our Worked Example), as the final answer may not appear obvious. But the following guide may be helpful in deciding whether your answer is reasonable or not.

The maximum you should give a patient:

Tablets: Not more than 4 for any one dose.*

Liquids: Anything from 5 ml to 20 ml for any one dose.

Injections: Anything from 1 ml to 10 ml for any one dose.

Any answer outside these ranges probably means that you have calculated the wrong answer.

---

* An exception to this would be prednisolone. Some doses of prednisolone may mean the patient taking up to 10 tablets at any one time. Even with prednisolone, it is important to check the dose and the number of tablets.

Re-check your answer. If you are in any doubt about any calculation – STOP and get help!

CALCULATION OF DRUG DOSAGES – SUMMARY

$$\frac{\text{Amount you want}}{\text{Amount you've got}} \times \text{Volume it's in}$$

Before entering numbers in the formula, convert everything to the same units, i.e.

Work in grams (g)

or

in milligrams (mg)

or

in micrograms (mcg)

or

Whatever units you are working in

PROBLEMS

B.11 You need to give a slow I.V. injection of salbutamol 250 mcg. Salbutamol injection comes as a 50 mcg/ml ampoule. How many ml do you need to draw up?

B.12 You have an ampoule of potassium chloride injection 1 g in 5 ml. The amount required equals 400 mg. How many ml do you need to draw up?

B.13 You need to give 1 g of erythromycin orally. You have erythromycin suspension 250 mg in 5 ml. How much of the suspension do you need to give?

B.14 You need to give 1 g of nalidixic acid orally. You have nalidixic acid suspension 300 mg in 5 ml. How much of the suspension do you give?

B.15 You need to give a slow I.V. injection of aminophylline 325 mg. Aminophylline injection comes as 250 mg in 10 ml ampoules. How many ml do you need to draw up?

B.16 You have an ampoule of potassium chloride injection 2 g in 10 ml. You need to add 1.8 g to a litre of sodium chloride 0.9% infusion. How much of the potassium chloride do you need?

B.17 You have to give phenytoin I.V. at a dose of 15 mg/kg. Phenytoin injection comes as 50 mg/ml ampoules and the patient weighs 73 kg. How much of the phenytoin injection do you need?

B.18 You need to give a dose of trimethoprim suspension to a child weighing 18.45 kg at a dose of 4 mg/kg. You have trimethoprim suspension 50 mg in 5 ml. What dose do you need to give and how much of the suspension do you need?

B.19 You have an injection of potassium chloride containing 27 mmol in 10 ml. You need to add 15 mmol to an infusion. How much of the potassium chloride injection do you need to draw up?

B.20 You need to give an injection of heparin 12,500 units. You have heparin 5,000 units in 1 ml. How many ampoules do you need and how much do you need to draw up?

B.21 You have to give cefotaxime I.V. to a baby weighing 5.6 kg at a dose of 100 mg/kg/day in four divided doses. You have 500 mg vials of cefotaxime injection, and each vial has to be reconstituted to 2 ml. How much do you need for each dose?

B.22 You need to prepare an infusion of co-trimoxazole at a dose of 120 mg/kg/day in four divided doses for a patient weighing 68 kg. Co-trimoxazole comes as 5 ml ampoules at a strength of 96 mg/ml.

(a) What volume of co-trimoxazole do you need for each dose?

(b) How many ampoules do you need for each dose?

(c) How many ampoules do you need for 24 hours?

(d) Before administration, co-trimoxazole must be diluted further: 1 ampoule diluted to 125 ml. Therefore what volume should each dose be given in?

ANSWERS TO PROBLEMS

B.1 Dose = 1.5 mg/kg, patient's weight = 73 kg. Therefore to calculate the total dose required, multiply:

$$1.5 \times 73 = 109.5$$

Thus you will need 109.5 mg (rounding up = 110 mg)

B.2 516 mg

B.3 720 mg

B.4 24.8 ml (25 ml)

B.5 97 mg

B.6 186 mg

B.7 (i) 21,600 mcg
(ii) 21.6 mg (22 mg)

B.8 325 mcg/min

B.9 255 mcg/min

B.10 $500 \times 78 = 39,000$ mcg/min

$$\frac{39,000}{1,000} = 39 \text{ mg/min}$$

B.11 5 ml

B.12 2 ml

B.13 20 ml

B.14 16.67 ml (17 ml)

B.15 13 ml

B.16 9 ml

B.17 Total amount required = Weight × Dose

$$= 73 \times 15 = 1{,}095 \text{ mg}$$

Volume required = 21.9 ml (22 ml)

B.18 Total amount required = Weight × Dose

$$= 18.45 \times 4 = 73.8 \text{ mg}$$

Volume required = 7.4 ml

B.19 You have an injection of potassium chloride containing 27 mmol in 10 ml. Calculate the volume for 1 mmol:

$$1 \text{ mmol} = \frac{10}{27} \text{ ml}$$

(you are using the '**one** unit' rule).

However, you need 15 mmol, therefore multiply the volume for 1 mmol by 15:

$$15 \text{ mmol} = \frac{10}{27} \times 15 = 5.55 \text{ ml } (5.5 \text{ ml approx.})$$

Or by using the formula

$$\frac{\text{Amount you want}}{\text{Amount you've got}} \times \text{Volume it's in}$$

where in this case:

Amount you want = 15 mmol
Amount you've got = 27 mmol
Volume it's in = 10 ml

substitute the numbers in the formula:

$$\frac{15}{27} \times 10 = 5.55 \text{ ml } (5.5 \text{ ml approx.})$$

B.20 You will need three 1 ml ampoules and to draw up 2.5 ml

B.21 Total daily dose = Weight × Dose
= 5.6 × 100 = 560 mg

This needs to be given in 4 divided doses, therefore to find out the amount needed for each dose, divide by 4:

$$\frac{560}{4} = 140\,\text{mg}$$

You have cefotaxime 500 mg in 2 ml. Thus

$$1\,\text{mg} = \frac{2}{500}\,\text{ml}$$

Therefore for 140 mg, you will need:

$$\frac{2}{500} \times 140 = 0.56\,\text{ml}$$

Or by using the formula

$$\frac{\text{Amount you want}}{\text{Amount you've got}} \times \text{Volume it's in}$$

where in this case:

Amount you want = 140 mg
Amount you've got = 500 mg
Volume it's in = 2 ml

substitute the numbers in the formula:

$$\frac{140}{500} \times 2 = 0.56\,\text{ml}$$

B.22 (a) Total daily dose = Weight × Dose
= 68 × 120 = 8,160 mg

However, this is to be given in 4 divided doses.
Therefore for each dose, you will need:

$$\frac{8,160}{4} = 2,040\,\text{mg}$$

You have co-trimoxazole injection containing 96 mg/ml. Thus

$$1 \, mg = \frac{1}{96} \, ml$$

Therefore for 2,040 mg you will need:

$$\frac{1}{96} \times 2{,}040 = 21.25 \, ml$$

(b) Each ampoule equals 5 ml. To work out how many ampoules are needed, divide the total volume required by the volume for each ampoule, i.e.

$$\frac{21.25}{5} = 4.25$$

Therefore you will need 5 ampoules (25 ml) for each dose, drawing up 21.25 ml and discarding the remainder.

(c) Since it is to be given in 4 divided doses, to calculate how many ampoules are needed for 1 day, multiply the amount for each dose by 4, i.e.

$$5 \times 4 = 20 \, ampoules$$

(d) 1 ampoule must be diluted to 125 ml, thus for 4.25 ampoules, you will need:

$$4.25 \times 125 = 531.25 \, ml$$

Therefore give in 1 litre sodium chloride infusion 0.9%.

5 Percent and percentages

INTRODUCTION

The percent or percentage is a common way of expressing the amount of something, and is very useful for comparing different quantities.

It is unlikely that you will need to calculate the percentage of something on the ward; it is more likely that you will need to know how much drug is in a solution given as a percentage, e.g. an infusion containing potassium 0.3%.

PERCENT AND PERCENTAGES

A convenient way of expressing drug strengths is by using the percent.

We will be dealing with how percentages are used to describe drug strengths or concentrations in Section 6 (Drug strengths or concentrations).

The aim of the present section is to explain the concept of percent and how to do simple percentage calculations.

> *Percent means 'part of a hundred' or 'proportion of a hundred'*

The symbol for percent is %. So 30% means 30 parts or units of 100.

Percent is often used to give a quick indication of a specific quantity and is very useful when making comparisons.

If you consider a town where 5,690 people live and the unemployment numbers are 853, it is very difficult to visualise exactly how many or what proportion of people are unemployed. It is much easier to say that in a town of 5,690 people, 15% of them are unemployed. Similarly, it is easier to compare numbers or quantities when given as percentages.

If we consider another town of 11,230 people where 2,246 people are unemployed, it is very difficult, at a glance, to see which town has the greater proportion of unemployed.

But when the numbers are given as percentages, it is much easier to compare: the first town has 15% unemployment, whereas the second town has 20% unemployed.

Thus, it can be seen that percentages can be very useful, and so is knowing how to convert to a percentage.

CONVERTING FRACTIONS TO PERCENTAGES AND VICE VERSA

To convert a fraction to a percentage, you simply **multiply** by 100, i.e.

$$\frac{2}{5} = \frac{2}{5} \times 100 = 40\%$$

Conversely, to convert a percentage to a fraction, **divide** by 100, i.e.

$$\frac{40}{100} = \frac{4}{10} = \frac{2}{5}$$

Always reduce the fraction to its lowest terms (if possible).

CONVERTING DECIMALS TO PERCENTAGES AND VICE VERSA

To convert a decimal to a percentage, you simply **multiply** by 100, i.e.

$$0.4 = 0.4 \times 100 = 40\%$$

You move the decimal point **two** places to the **right**.

Once again, if you want to convert a percentage to a decimal, you **divide** by 100, i.e.

$$\frac{40}{100} = 0.4$$

You move the decimal point **two** places to the **left**.

So, in conclusion, to convert fractions and decimals to percentages and vice versa, you simply multiply or divide by 100. Thus:

$$25\% = \frac{25}{100} = \frac{1}{4} = 0.25 \quad \text{(a quarter)}$$

$$33\% = \frac{33}{100} = \frac{1}{3} = 0.33 \quad \text{(about a third)}$$

$$50\% = \frac{50}{100} = \frac{1}{2} = 0.5 \quad \text{(a half)}$$

$$66\% = \frac{66}{100} = \frac{2}{3} = 0.66 \quad \text{(about two-thirds)}$$

$$75\% = \frac{75}{100} = \frac{3}{4} = 0.75 \quad \text{(three-quarters)}$$

CALCULATIONS INVOLVING PERCENTAGES

The first type of calculation we are going to look at is how to find the percentage of a given quantity or number. Hopefully, the following worked example will show how this is done.

WORKED EXAMPLE

How much is 28% of 250?

There are several ways of solving this type of calculation.

Method One
With this method you are working in percentages.

Step 1
When doing percentage calculations, the number or quantity you want to find the percentage of, is always equal to 100%.

In this example, 250 is equal to 100% and you want to find out how much is 28%. So,

$$250 = 100\%$$

(thus you are converting the number to a percentage).

Step 2
Calculate how much is equal to 1%, i.e. divide by 100:

$$1\% = \frac{250}{100}$$

(you are using the '**one** unit' rule).

Step 3
Multiply by the percentage required (28%):

$$28\% = \frac{250}{100} \times 28 = 70$$

Answer: 28% of 250 = 70.

Method Two
In this method you are working in either fractions or decimals and not percentages.

Step 1
To convert the percentage to a fraction or decimal, divide by 100, i.e.

$$\frac{28}{100} \quad \text{or} \quad 0.28$$

Step 2
Multiply by the number (250):

$$\frac{28}{100} \times 250 = 70$$

which is the same as:

$$0.28 \times 250 = 70$$

Thus you are finding out how much the fraction or decimal is of the original number.

Answer: 28% of 250 = 70.

From both methods used, a simple formula can be devised:

$$\frac{\textbf{Number}}{\textbf{100}} \times \textbf{Percentage required}$$

In this example:

Number $= 250$

Percentage required $= 28\%$

Substitute the numbers in the formula:

$$\frac{250}{100} \times 28 = 70$$

Answer: 28% of 250 = 70.

Note that whatever method you use, you always **divide by 100.**

However, you may want to find out what percentage a number is of another larger number, especially when comparing numbers or quantities. So this is the second type of percentage calculation we are going to look at.

WORKED EXAMPLE

What percentage is 630 of 9,000?

In this case, it is best to work in percentages since it is a percentage that you want to find.

Step 1
Once again, the number or quantity you want to find the percentage of, is always equal to 100%.

In this example, 9,000 is equal to 100% and you want to find out the percentage of 630. So,

$$9,000 = 100\%$$

(thus you are converting the number to a percentage).

Step 2
Calculate the percentage for 1, i.e. divide by 9,000:

$$\frac{100}{9,000}\%$$

(you are using the '**one** unit' rule).

Step 3
Multiply by the number you wish to find the percentage of, i.e. the smaller number (630):

$$\frac{100}{9,000} \times 630 = 7\%$$

Answer: 630 is 7% of 9,000.

Once again, a simple formula can be devised:

$$\frac{100}{\textbf{Larger number}} \times \frac{\textbf{Smaller}}{\textbf{number}} \quad \text{or} \quad \frac{\textbf{Smaller number}}{\textbf{Larger number}} \times \textbf{100}$$

Note that in this case, you **multiply by 100** (it is always on the top line).

PERCENT AND PERCENTAGES – SUMMARY

> To convert a fraction to a percentage, **multiply** by 100

To convert a percentage to a fraction, **divide** by 100

To convert a decimal to a percentage, **multiply** by 100
You move the decimal point **two** places to the **right**

To convert a percentage to a decimal, **divide** by 100
You move the decimal point **two** places to the **left**

How to find the percentage of a number:

$$\frac{\text{Number}}{100} \times \text{Percentage required}$$

Note: Always **divide** by 100.

How to find what percentage one number is of another:

$$\frac{100}{\text{Larger number}} \times \text{Smaller number} \quad \text{or} \quad \frac{\text{Smaller number}}{\text{Larger number}} \times 100$$

Note: Always **multiply** by 100.

PROBLEMS

Work out the following:

C.1 30% of 3,090
C.2 84% of 42,825
C.3 56.25% of 800
C.4 60% of 80.6
C.5 17.5% of 285.76

What percentage are the following?
C.6 60 of 750
C.7 53,865 of 64,125
C.8 29.61 of 47
C.9 53.69 of 191.75
C.10 48 of 142

DRUG CALCULATIONS INVOLVING PERCENTAGES

The principles here can easily be applied to drug calculations.

As before, it is unlikely that you will need to find the percentage of something, but these calculations are included here in order to gain an understanding of percent and percentages, especially where drugs are concerned.

Once again, always convert everything to the same units before solving the calculation.

WORKED EXAMPLE

How many ml is 60% of 1.25 litres?

(This is similar to the first type of calculation.)

Step 1
Convert 1.25 litres into millilitres (ml), since the required answer is in millilitres (ml), i.e.

$$1.25 \text{ litres} = 1.25 \times 1{,}000 = 1{,}250 \text{ ml}$$

Step 2
As before, the quantity you want to find the percentage of is always equal to 100%, i.e.

$$1{,}250 \text{ ml} = 100\%$$

Thus you are converting the volume to a percentage.

Step 3
Calculate how many ml equals 1% by dividing by 100:

$$1\% = \frac{1{,}250}{100}$$

(using the '**one** unit' rule).

Step 4
Multiply by the percentage required (60%):

$$60\% = \frac{1{,}250}{100} \times 60 = 750 \text{ ml}$$

Answer: 60% of 1.25 litres equals 750 ml.

Alternatively, you can use the formula:

$$\frac{\text{Number}}{100} \times \text{Percentage required}$$

Rewrite it as:

$$\frac{\text{What you've got}}{100} \times \text{Percentage required}$$

where

What you've got = 1,250 ml

Percentage required = 60%

Substitute the numbers in the formula:

$$\frac{1,250}{100} \times 60 = 750 \text{ ml}$$

Answer: 60% of 1.25 litres is 750 ml.

Now consider the following:

WORKED EXAMPLE

What percentage is 125 mg of 500 mg?

Step 1
Always convert everything to the same units. In this case, everything is in milligrams (mg), so it is not necessary to convert to the same units.

If you were working in different units, convert everything to the same units (usually those of the answer, but *always* to the units that avoid decimal points).

Step 2
As always, the quantity you want to find the percentage of is equal to 100%, i.e.

500 mg = 100%

Thus you are converting the quantity or amount to a percentage.

Step 3

Calculate the percentage for 1 mg of what you have by dividing by 500, i.e.

$$1 \text{ mg} = \frac{100}{500} \%$$

(you are using the '**one** unit' rule).

Step 4

However, you want to know the percentage for 125 mg, thus multiply by 125 mg, i.e.

$$125 \text{ mg} = \frac{100}{500} \times 125 = 25\%$$

Answer: 125 mg is equal to 25% of 500 mg.

Alternatively, you can use the formula:

$$\frac{100}{\text{Larger number}} \times \text{Smaller number}$$

where:

> Smaller number = 125 mg
> Larger number = 500 mg

Substitute the numbers in the formula:

$$\frac{100}{500} \times 125 = 25\%$$

Answer: 125 mg is equal to 25% of 500 mg.

From these calculations, you would have noticed that the higher the percentage, the stronger the solution. Thus, a 20% solution is stronger than a 15% solution.

DRUG CALCULATIONS INVOLVING PERCENTAGES – SUMMARY

How to find the percentage of something:

$$\frac{\text{What you've got}}{100} \times \text{Percentage required}$$

How to find what percentage one quantity is of another:

$$\frac{100}{\text{Larger number}} \times \text{Smaller number}$$

PROBLEMS

Work out the following:

C.11 How much is 15% of 3 litres?
C.12 How much is 63% of 2.5 litres?
C.13 How much is 28% of 500 g?
C.14 How much is 98% of 3 kg?
C.15 How much is 27.6% of 500 ml?

What percentage are the following?
C.16 230 ml of 500 ml
C.17 48 g of 750 g
C.18 320 mg of 800 mg
C.19 64.5 g of 250 g
C.20 750 mg of 5 g N.B. Beware of units
C.21 64.5 mg of 1 g N.B. Beware of units

HOW TO USE THE PERCENTAGE KEY ON YOUR CALCULATOR

A quick way to work out percentages is to use the [%] button on your calculator. However, it is important that the numbers and the [%] button are pressed in the right sequence, otherwise you will get the wrong answer! N.B. Your calculator may show a different display to those shown here.

Let us go back to our original example:

How much is 28% of 250?

You could easily find the answer by the long method, i.e.

$$\frac{250}{100} \times 28$$

Key in the sequence: [2] [5] [0] [÷] [1] [0] [0] [×] [2] [8] [=], to give an answer of 70.

But when using the [%] button, you need to enter in the following way:

ENTER	[2] [8]	DISPLAY = 28
ENTER	[×]	DISPLAY = 28
ENTER	[2] [5] [0]	DISPLAY = 250
ENTER	[%]	DISPLAY = 70 (answer)
ENTER	[=]	DISPLAY = 1960

Depending upon which calculator you have, pressing the [=] may give the wrong answer! What happens in such cases is that by pressing the [=] button, you are multiplying by the percentage again, i.e.

28 × 28% of 250

giving a nonsensical answer!

Let us now look at the second example:

What percentage is 630 of 9,000?

Once again, you can easily find the answer by

$$\frac{630}{9,000} \times 100$$

Key in the sequence [6] [3] [0] [÷] [9] [0] [0] [0] [×] [1] [0] [0] [=] to give an answer of 7.

But when using the [%] button, you need to enter in the following way:

ENTER	[6] [3] [0]	DISPLAY = 630
ENTER	[÷]	DISPLAY = 630
ENTER	[9] [0] [0] [0]	DISPLAY = 9000
ENTER	[%]	DISPLAY = 7 (answer)
ENTER	[=]	DISPLAY = 0.07777

Once again, pressing the [=] may give the wrong answer! What happens is that by pressing the [=] button, you are dividing by 9,000 again, i.e.

$$\frac{630}{9,000 \times 9,000} \times 100$$

Thus when using your calculator, **do not press the [=] button**.

It is important to enter the numbers in the right sequence; if not, you will again get the wrong answer:

ENTER	[9] [0] [0] [0]	DISPLAY = 9000
ENTER	[÷]	DISPLAY = 9000
ENTER	[6] [3] [0]	DISPLAY = 630
ENTER	[%]	DISPLAY = 1428.5714

If you enter [=]

| ENTER | [=] | DISPLAY = 2.2675736 |

To explain this, let us look at the long method of solving this problem:

$$9,000 = 100\%$$

Therefore

$$1 = \frac{100}{9,000} \%$$

Thus

$$630 = \frac{100}{9,000} \times 630\% \text{ or } \frac{630}{9,000} \times 100\%$$

You can see that it is 630 *divided* by 9,000, and not the other way round.

Therefore it is important to enter the numbers the right way round on your calculator.

An easy way to remember which way round to enter the numbers is: enter the *smaller* number *first*.

It is also important to remember to enter or press the [%] button *last*, otherwise you will get the wrong answer, i.e. in our first example: How much is 28% of 250?

ENTER	[2] [8]	DISPLAY = 28
ENTER	[%]	DISPLAY = 28
ENTER	[×]	DISPLAY = 28
ENTER	[2] [5] [0]	DISPLAY = 250
ENTER	[=]	DISPLAY = 7000

You are simply multiplying 28 by 250.

In both examples, entering the numbers in the wrong sequence will give the wrong answer. Try experimenting with your own calculator; you will soon see how many different answers you can get!

So, to summarise, if you want to use the [%] button on your calculator, remember the following sequence:

1. Enter the numbers in the right sequence.
   If you are finding the percentage of something: **multiply** the two numbers (it doesn't matter in which order you enter the numbers).
   If you are find the percentage one number is of another: **divide** the **smaller** number (enter *first*) by the **larger** number (enter *second*). In this case, the sequence of numbers is important.
2. Always enter or press the [%] button *last*.
3. Do *not* enter or press the [=] button.
4. Refer to your calculator manual to see how your own calculator uses the [%] button.
5. Don't forget to clear your calculator (press the [CE] button), otherwise the numbers left in your calculator may be carried over to your next sum.

Although using the [%] button is a quick way of finding percentages, you have to use it properly. If you are unsure, do the calculations the long way.

ANSWERS TO PROBLEMS

Calculations involving percentages

C.1 927
C.2 35,973

C.3 450

C.4 48.36

C.5 50.008 (50)

C.6 8%

C.7 84%

C.8 63%

C.9 28%

C.10 33.8%

Drug calculations involving percentages

C.11 0.45 litres (450 ml)

C.12 1.575 litres (1,575 ml)

C.13 140 g

C.14 2.94 kg (2,940 g)

C.15 138 ml

C.16 46%

C.17 6.4%

C.18 40%

C.19 25.8%

C.20 It is best to work in whole numbers, so convert the larger unit (grams) to the smaller unit (milligrams):

$$5 \times 1,000 = 5,000 \, \text{mg}$$
$$5,000 \, \text{mg} = 100\%$$

thus

$$1 \, \text{mg} = \frac{100}{5,000} \, \%$$

Therefore

$$750 \, \text{mg} = \frac{100}{5,000} \times 750 = 15\%$$

Answer: 750 mg is 15% of 5 g.

If using the formula:

$$\frac{100}{\text{Larger number}} \times \text{Smaller number}$$

where:

> Smaller number = 750 mg
> Larger number = 5,000 mg (5 g)

(always work in the *same* units – in this case it is best to work in milligrams since this is the smaller unit), substitute the numbers in the formula:

$$\frac{100}{5,000} \times 750 = 15\%$$

Answer: 750 mg is 15% of 5 g.

C.21 Beware of units; convert 1 g to 1,000 mg.

> *Answer:* 6.45%.

Drug strengths or concentrations
6

OBJECTIVES

At the end of this section, you should be familiar with the following:

Percentage concentration
  To calculate the total amount of drug in a solution
  To calculate dosages from percentage concentrations
mg/ml concentrations

To convert percentages to a mg/ml concentration
To convert mg/ml concentrations to a percentage
'1 in ...' concentrations or ratio strengths
Tuberculin strengths
Drugs with units: heparin and insulin

INTRODUCTION

There are various ways of expressing how much actual drug is present in a medicine. These medicines are usually liquids that are for oral or parenteral administration, but also include those for topical use.

The aim of this section is to explain the various ways in which drug strengths can be stated.

PERCENTAGE CONCENTRATION

Following on from the last section, one method of describing concentration is to use the percentage as a unit.

The most common one you will come across is the percentage concentration, w/v (weight in volume). This is when a solid is

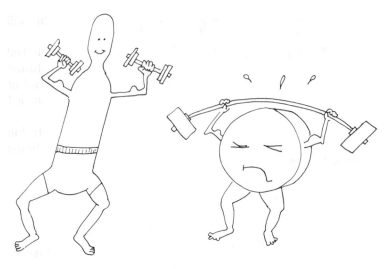

Drug strengths

dissolved in a liquid and means the number of grams dissolved in 100 ml.

% w/v = number of grams in 100 ml
(Thus 5% w/v means 5 g in 100 ml)

Another type of concentration you might come across is the percentage concentration, w/w (weight in weight). This is when a solid is mixed with another solid, e.g. creams and ointments, and means the number of grams in 100 g.

% w/w = number of grams in 100 g
(Thus 5% w/w means 5 g in 100 g)

Another concentration is the percentage concentration, v/v (volume in volume). This is when a liquid is mixed or diluted with another liquid, and means the number of ml in 100 ml.

% v/v = number of millilitres in 100 ml
(Thus 5% v/v means 5 ml in 100 ml)

The most common percentage concentration you will encounter is the percentage w/v or 'weight in volume' and therefore this will be the one considered here.

Thus in our earlier example of 5% w/v, there are 5 g in 100 ml irrespective of the size of the container, e.g. dextrose 5% infusion means that there are 5 g of dextrose dissolved in each 100 ml of fluid and this will remain the same if there is a 500 ml bag or a 1 litre bag.

To find the total amount of drug present in a bottle or infusion bag, you must take into account the size or volume of the bottle or infusion bag.

WORKED EXAMPLE

To calculate the total amount of drug in a solution

How much sodium bicarbonate is there in a 200 ml infusion of sodium bicarbonate 8.4% w/v?

Step 1
Convert the percentage to the number of grams in 100 ml, i.e.

> 8.4% = 8.4 g in 100 ml

(You are converting the percentage to a specific quantity.)

Step 2
Calculate how many grams there are in 1 ml, i.e. divide by 100:

$$\frac{8.4}{100} \text{ g in 1 ml}$$

(using the '**one** unit' rule).

Step 3
However, you have a 200 ml infusion. So to find out the total amount present, multiply how much is in 1 ml by the volume you've got (200 ml):

$$\frac{8.4}{100} \times 200 = 16.8 \text{ g in 200 ml}$$

Answer: There are 16.8 g of sodium bicarbonate in 200 ml of sodium bicarbonate 8.4% w/v infusion.

A simple formula can be devised based upon a formula seen earlier:

$$\frac{\text{Number}}{100} \times \text{Percentage required}$$

This can be rearranged to give:

$$\frac{\text{Percentage}}{100} \times \text{Number}$$

where

Percentage = The percentage of what you've got
Number = Total volume you've got

Therefore it can be rewritten as:

$$\text{Total amount in g} = \frac{\text{Percentage}}{100} \times \text{Total volume in ml}$$

Therefore in the Worked Example:

Percentage   = 8.4%
Total volume in ml = 200 ml

Substituting the numbers in the formula:

$$\text{Total amount in g} = \frac{8.4}{100} \times 200 = 16.8 \, \text{g}$$

Answer: There are 16.8 g of sodium bicarbonate in 200 ml of sodium bicarbonate 8.4% w/v infusion.

Once again, the type of calculations seen with percentage concentrations are similar to the ones seen earlier.

WORKED EXAMPLE

To calculate dosages from percentage concentrations

You have salbutamol nebuliser solution 0.5%. What volume is required for a 2.5 mg dose?

Step 1
Write down what 0.5% exactly represents; 0.5% means:

0.5 g in 100 ml

Step 2
Convert 0.5 g to mg by multiplying by 1,000 (the dose required is in mg):

$$0.5 \text{ g} = 0.5 \times 1,000 = 500 \text{ mg}$$

Step 3
Of what you've got, work out the volume for 1 mg, thus:

500 mg in 100 ml

$$1 \text{ mg} = \frac{100}{500} \text{ ml}$$

(using the 'one' unit' rule).

Step 4
Now work out the volume required for the dose needed, i.e.

$$2.5 \text{ mg} = \frac{100}{500} \times 2.5 = 0.5 \text{ ml}$$

Answer: The volume required = 0.5 ml

Alternatively, you can use a formula you have met earlier when calculating drug dosages:

$$\frac{\text{Amount you want}}{\text{Amount you've got}} \times \text{Volume it's in}$$

Once again, before substituting numbers in the formula, convert everything to the same units. Thus:

0.5% = 0.5 g in 100 ml
   or   500 mg in 100 ml

In this situation, the 'Volume it's in' is therefore 100 ml.

There is no need to worry about the volume of the bottle, ampoule or whatever.

Always convert the percentage to an amount in 100 ml. Therefore the formula can be rewritten as:

$$\frac{\text{Amount you want}}{\text{Amount you've got}} \times 100$$

So:

Amount you want $= 2.5\,\text{mg}$
Amount you've got $= 500\,\text{mg}$

Substituting the numbers in the formula:

$$\frac{2.5}{500} \times 100 = 0.5\,\text{ml}$$

Answer: The volume required $= 0.5\,\text{ml}$.

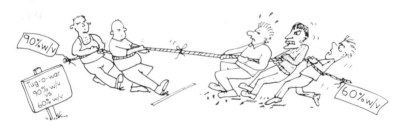

PERCENTAGE CONCENTRATION – SUMMARY

Percentage 'weight in volume' (% w/v):

> % w/v = number of grams per 100 ml

Percentage 'weight in weight' (% w/w):

> % w/v = number of grams per 100 g

Percentage 'volume in volume' (% v/v):

> % w/v = number of millilitres per 100 ml

PROBLEMS

D.1 How many grams of sodium chloride are there in a litre infusion of sodium chloride 0.9%?

D.2 How many grams of potassium, sodium and glucose are there in a litre infusion of potassium 0.3%, sodium chloride 0.18% and glucose 4%?

D.3 How many grams of sodium chloride are there in a 500 ml infusion of sodium chloride 0.45%?

D.4 You need to give a continuous infusion containing calcium gluconate 4 g. You have 10 ml ampoules of calcium gluconate 10%. How much do you need to draw up?

D.5 You need to give a dose of 200 mg of chloral hydrate to a child. You have a bottle of chloral hydrate (paediatric) 4%. What volume do you give?

D.6 You need to add 1.5 g of potassium chloride to 500 ml of sodium chloride 0.9%. You have 5 ml ampoules of 10% potassium chloride. What volume of potassium chloride do you need to draw up?

mg/ml CONCENTRATIONS

Another way of expressing the amount or concentration of drug in a solution, usually for oral or parenteral administration, is mg/ml, i.e. number of mg of drug per ml of liquid.

This is the most common way of expressing the amount of drug in a solution.

For oral liquids, it is usually expressed as the number of mg in a standard 5 ml spoonful, e.g. erythromycin 250 mg in 5 ml.

For injections, it is usually expressed as the number of mg per volume of the ampoule (1 ml, 2 ml, 5 ml, 10 ml and 20 ml), e.g. frusemide 10 mg/ml and gentamicin 80 mg in 2 ml.

Strengths can also be expressed in mcg/ml, e.g. hyoscine injection 600 mcg/ml. Only mg/ml will be considered here, but the principles learnt here can be applied to other concentrations or strengths, e.g. mcg/ml.

Sometimes it may be useful to convert percentage concentrations to mg/ml concentrations. For example:

Lignocaine 0.2%   = 0.2 g per 100 ml
                                   = 200 mg per 100 ml
                                   = 2 mg per ml (2 mg/ml)

Sodium chloride 0.9% = 0.9 g per 100 ml
                                   = 900 mg per 100 ml
                                   = 9 mg per ml (9 mg/ml)

Glucose 5%   = 5 g per 100 ml
                                   = 5,000 mg per 100 ml
                                   = 50 mg per ml (50 mg/ml)

This will give the strength of the solution irrespective of the size of the bottle, infusion bag, etc.

An easy way of finding the strength in mg/ml is by simply multiplying the percentage by 10. This can be explained using lignocaine 0.2% as an example:

You have lignocaine 0.2%. This is equal to 0.2 g in 100 ml. Divide by 100 to find out how much is in 1 ml. Thus:

$$\frac{0.2}{100} \text{ g/ml}$$

Multiply by 1,000 to convert grams to milligrams, thus:

$$\frac{0.2}{100} \times 1,000 \text{ mg/ml}$$

Simplify the above sum to give:

$$0.2 \times 10 = 2 \text{ mg/ml}$$

Therefore you simply multiply the percentage by 10.

With our earlier examples:

Lignocaine 0.2%   = 0.2 × 10 = 2 mg/ml
Sodium chloride 0.9% = 0.9 × 10 = 9 mg/ml
Glucose 5%   = 5   × 10 = 50 mg/ml

Consequently, to convert a mg/ml concentration to a percentage, you simply divide by 10.

Once again, if we use our original lignocaine as an example:

You have lignocaine 2 mg/ml. Percentage means 'per 100 ml', so multiply by 100, i.e.

$$2 \text{ mg/ml} \times 100 = 200 \text{ mg/100 ml} \ (2 \times 100)$$

Percentage (w/v) means 'the number of grams per 100 ml', so you will have to convert milligrams to grams by dividing by 1,000, i.e.

$$\frac{2 \times 100}{1,000} = \frac{2}{10} = 0.2\%$$

Therefore you simply divide the mg/ml concentration by 10.

With our earlier examples:

Lignocaine 2 mg/ml   = 2 ÷ 10 = 0.2%
Sodium chloride 9 mg/ml = 9 ÷ 10 = 0.9%
Glucose 50 mg/ml   = 50 ÷ 10 = 5%

Once again, calculations with mg/ml are the same as seen earlier with dosage calculations.

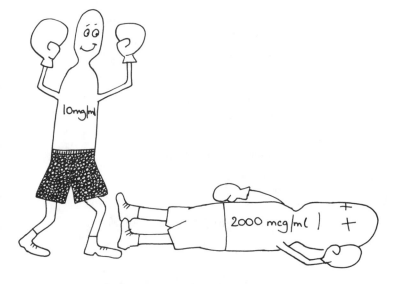

WORKED EXAMPLE

You have codeine phosphate syrup 25 mg in 5 ml. You need a dose of 30 mg; what volume do you give?

Step 1
Write down the strength you've got:

25 mg in 5 ml

Step 2
Calculate the volume for 1 mg:

$$1 \text{ mg} = \frac{5}{25} \text{ ml}$$

(using the '**one** unit' rule).

Step 3
Multiply by the dose required:

$$30 \text{ mg} = \frac{5}{25} \times 30 = 6 \text{ ml}$$

Answer: You will need 6 ml for a dose of 30 mg.

The formula seen earlier with calculating dosages can be used here:

$$\frac{\text{Amount you want}}{\text{Amount you've got}} = \text{Volume it's in}$$

where in this case:

Amount you want = 30 mg
Amount you've got = 25 mg
Volume it's in   = 5 ml

Substitute the numbers in the formula:

$$\frac{30}{25} \times 5 = 6 \text{ ml}$$

Answer: You will need 6 ml for a dose of 30 mg.

mg/ml **CONCENTRATIONS – SUMMARY**

> mg/ml = number of mg per 1 ml

> To convert a percentage to a mg/ml concentration –
> **multiply by 10**

> To convert a mg/ml concentration to a percentage –
> **divide by 10**

PROBLEMS

Calculate the strengths (mg/ml) for the following:

- **D.7** Sodium chloride infusion 0.45%
- **D.8** Metronidazole infusion 0.5%
- **D.9** Potassium chloride 0.2%, sodium chloride 0.18% and glucose 4%

Solve the following:

- **D.10** You have pethidine injection 100 mg in 2 ml. The patient is prescribed 75 mg. How much do you draw up?
- **D.11** You have morphine sulphate elixir 10 mg in 5 ml. The patient is prescribed 25 mg. How much do you give?
- **D.12** You have gentamicin injection 80 mg in 2 ml. The patient is prescribed 100 mg. How much do you need?

'1 IN ...' **CONCENTRATIONS OR RATIO STRENGTHS**

This final type of concentration is only used occasionally. It is written as '1 in ...', e.g. 1 in 10,000, and is sometimes known as a ratio strength.

It means **one** gram in however many ml. For example:

1 in 1,000 means 1 g in 1,000 ml
1 in 10,000 means 1 g in 10,000 ml

Therefore it can be seen that 1 in 10,000 is weaker than 1 in 1,000. So, the higher the 'number', the weaker the solution.

Tuberculin

The exception to this is tuberculin. Strengths are sometimes written in a '1 in . . .' notation. For example:

1 in 10,000   (10 units/ml)
1 in 1,000   (100 units/ml)
1 in 100   (1,000 units/ml)

It is *not* 1 g in 10,000 ml, etc., but is simply a dilution: 1 ml diluted 10,000 times.

So it is important that you don't get confused between the two notations.

Undiluted tuberculin contains 100,000 units per ml. A 1 in 10,000 dilution is therefore equal to:

$$\frac{100,000}{10,000} \text{ units/ml} = 10 \text{ units/ml}$$

(1 ml diluted 10,000 times). A 1 in 1,000 dilution is equal to:

$$\frac{100,000}{1,000} \text{ units/ml} = 100 \text{ units/ml}$$

(1 ml diluted 1,000 times). A 1 in 100 dilution is equal to:

$$\frac{100,000}{100} \text{ units/ml} = 1,000 \text{ unit/ml}$$

(1 ml diluted 100 times).

It is better to write the concentration as 10 U/ml instead of 1 in 10,000 to avoid confusion; but the old notation is still used.

'1 IN . . .' CONCENTRATIONS – SUMMARY

'1 in . . .' = 1 g in however many ml

HEPARIN AND INSULIN

The purity of drugs, such as insulin and heparin, from animal or biosynthetic sources varies. Therefore these drugs are expressed in terms of *units* as a standard measurement rather than weight.

Thus for heparin and insulin the following strengths are available:

Heparin	1,000 units/ml	1 ml, 5 ml, 10 ml ampoules
	5,000 units/ml	1 ml, 5 ml ampoules
	10,000 units/ml	1 ml ampoules
	25,000 units/ml	1 ml ampoules

N.B.There is a strength of 25,000 units/ml available for subcutaneous use as 0.2 ml ampoules containing 5,000 units.

| **Insulin** 100 units per ml | 10 ml vials |

Heparin

Heparin is given subcutaneously, two or three times a day, or by continuous intravenous infusion. Infusions are usually given over 24 hours and the dose is adjusted according to laboratory results. Therefore doses can vary, so it is important to know how to calculate how much heparin is needed.

Whatever the dose prescribed, you would choose the most appropriate ampoule(s) for that dose depending upon which strengths of heparin are available.

For example:

Dose = 28,000 units

You would choose:

1 × 25,000 units/ml ampoule *plus*
3 × 1,000 units/ml ampoule
(*or* 1 × 5,000 units/ml – using part of the ampoule)

As you can see, there are still some calculations involved with heparin dosages.

Calculations involving units are exactly the same as those seen earlier (see Section 4 on Dosage Calculations), but you are working in units instead of milligrams and micrograms.

WORKED EXAMPLE

You need to give heparin as a continuous infusion, 28,000 units in 48 ml normal saline over 24 hours.

Assuming that the only strengths of heparin available are 25,000 units/ml and 5,000 units/ml, how much do you need to draw up for the dose prescribed?

Step 1
In this case the dose = 28,000 units. Therefore you would use:

1 × 25,000 units/ml, 1 ml ampoule *plus*
1 × 5,000 units/ml, 1 ml ampoule

N.B. If 1,000 units/ml ampoules were available, then you would use 3 × 1,000 units/ml instead.

Step 2
Calculate how much of the 5,000 units/ml ampoule you need:

28,000 units − 25,000 units = 3,000 units

Therefore you need to draw up 3,000 units from the 5,000 units/ml ampoule.

Step 3
Write down what you have, i.e.

5,000 units in 1 ml

Step 4
Work out the volume for 1 unit:

5,000 units in 1 ml

$$1 \text{ unit} = \frac{1}{5,000} \text{ ml}$$

(using the '**one** unit' rule).

Step 5
Now multiply by the dose required (3,000 units):

$$3,000 \text{ units} = \frac{1}{5,000} \times 3,000 = 0.6 \text{ ml}$$

Answer: You would add 1 × 25,000 units/ml ampoule and 0.6 ml of 1 × 5,000 units/ml to the infusion.

Alternatively, you could use the formula seen earlier in Section 4 on Dosage calculations:

$$\frac{\text{Amount you want}}{\text{Amount you've got}} \times \text{Volume it's in}$$

Once again, before substituting numbers in the formula, decide as to which ampoule(s) of heparin would be the most appropriate; then, if necessary, calculate how much to draw up. Thus:

Amount you want   = 3,000 units
Amount you've got = 5,000 units
Volume it's in   = 1 ml

Substitute the numbers in the formula:

$$\frac{3,000}{5,000} \times 1 = 0.6 \text{ ml}$$

Answer: You would add 1 × 25,000 units/ml ampoule and 0.6 ml of 1 × 5,000 units/ml to the infusion.

Insulin

There are no calculations involved in the administration of insulin. Insulin comes in vials containing 100 units, and the doses prescribed are written in units.

Therefore, all you have to do is to draw up the required dose using an insulin syringe.

Insulin syringes are calibrated as 100 units in 1 ml and are available as 1 ml and 0.5 ml syringes.

So if the dose is 30 units, you simply draw up to the 30 unit mark on the syringe.

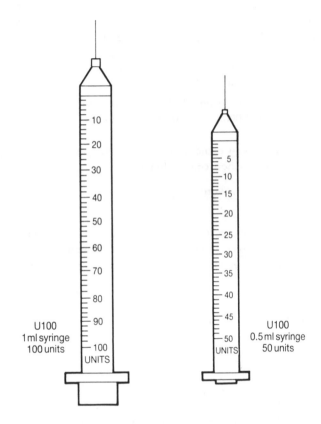

FIGURE 6.1 Actual size insulin U100 syringes.

PROBLEMS

D.13 Adrenaline is sometimes combined with lignocaine when used as a local anaesthetic, usually as a 1 in 200,000 strength. How much adrenaline is there in a 20 ml vial?

D.14 Sometimes adrenaline eye drops may be written as: adrenaline 1 in 100. What percentage strength is this?

D.15 You need to give an infusion of heparin containing 27,000 units over 24 hours. Assuming that the only strengths available are 25,000 units/ml and 5,000 units/ml, how much do you need to draw up for the dose prescribed?

D.16 You need to give an infusion of heparin containing 29,000 units over 24 hours. Assuming that the only strengths available are 25,000 units/ml and 5,000 units/ml, how much do you need to draw up for the dose prescribed?

ANSWERS TO PROBLEMS

D.1 0.9 g in 100 ml
9 g in 1,000 ml

D.2 Potassium   0.3 g in 100 ml
                3 g in 1,000 ml
       Sodium   0.18 g in 100 ml
                1.8 g in 1,000 ml
       Glucose   4 g in 100 ml
                40 g in 1,000 ml

D.3 0.45 g in 100 ml
2.25 g in 500 ml

D.4 Calcium gluconate 10% is equal to:

10 g in 100 ml

Therefore in a 10 ml ampoule, there is 1 g calcium gluconate. But you need 4 g, i.e. 4 ampoules = 4 g or 40 ml calcium gluconate 10%.

If using the formula:

$$\frac{\text{Amount you want}}{\text{Amount you've got}} \times 100$$

where in this case:

Amount you want   = 4 g
Amount you've got = 10 g (10% = 10 g in 100 ml)

(everything is in the same units, so there is no need to change units), substitute the numbers in the formula:

$$\frac{4}{10} \times 100 = 40 \text{ ml}$$

Answer: You need to draw up 40 ml, which is equivalent to 4 ampoules.

D.5 Chloral hydrate 4% is equal to:

4 g in 100 ml

Convert to milligrams (dose is in milligrams) to give 4,000 mg in 100 ml.

Work out the volume for 1 mg of what you've got, i.e. 4,000 mg in 100 ml:

$$1 \text{ mg in } \frac{100}{4,000} \text{ ml}$$

(using the 'one unit' rule).

Now multiply by the dose required (200 mg), i.e.

$$200 \text{ mg} = \frac{100}{4,000} \times 200 = 5 \text{ ml}$$

Or use the formula:

$$\frac{\text{Amount you want}}{\text{Amount you've got}} \times 100$$

where in this case:

Amount you want = 200 mg
Amount you've got = 4 g (4% = 4 g in 100 ml)

Before putting the numbers into the formula, convert everything to the same units. In this case, convert to milligrams: the dose required is in milligrams. Thus:

4 g = 4 × 1,000 = 4,000 mg
Amount you've got = 4,000 mg

Substitute the numbers in the formula:

$$\frac{200}{4,000} \times 100 = 5 \text{ ml}$$

Answer: You need to give 5 ml for a dose of 200 mg.

D.6 Potassium chloride is equal to:

10 g in 100 ml

However, you have a 5 ml ampoule. Work out how much is in 1 ml:

$$1\,\text{ml} = \frac{10}{100}\,\text{g}$$

(using the '**one** unit' rule).

Now multiply by the volume of the ampoule (5 ml):

$$5\,\text{ml} = \frac{10}{100} \times 5 = 0.5\,\text{g}$$

Therefore each 5 ml ampoule contains 0.5 g of potassium. Thus for your dose of 1.5 g, you will need to draw up 3 ampoules or 15 ml.

Answer: You need to draw up 15 ml, which is equivalent to 3 ampoules.

If using the formula:

$$\frac{\text{Amount you want}}{\text{Amount you've got}} \times 100$$

where in this case:

Amount you want   = 1.5 g
Amount you've got = 10 g ($10\% = 10$ g in 100 ml)

(everything is in the same units, so there is no need to change units), substitute the numbers in the formula:

$$\frac{1.5}{10} \times 100 = 15\,\text{ml}$$

Answer: You need to draw up 15 ml, which is equivalent to 3 ampoules.

D.7 4.5 mg/ml
D.8 5 mg/ml
D.9 Potassium   2 mg/ml
Sodium chloride 1.8 mg/ml
Glucose   40 mg/ml
D.10 You have pethidine 100 mg in 2 ml. Work out how much 1 mg is:

100 mg in 2 ml

$$1 \, \text{mg in} \, \frac{2}{100} \, \text{ml}$$

(using the '**one** unit' rule).

Now multiply by the dose required (75 mg):

$$75 \, \text{mg} = \frac{2}{100} \times 75 = 1.5 \, \text{ml}$$

Answer: You need to draw up 1.5 ml.

If using the formula:

$$\frac{\text{Amount you want}}{\text{Amount you've got}} \times \text{Volume it's in}$$

where in this case:

Amount you want   = 75 mg
Amount you've got = 100 mg
Volume it's in   = 2 ml

substitute the numbers in the formula:

$$\frac{75}{100} \times 2 = 1.5 \, \text{ml}$$

Answer: You need to draw up 1.5 ml.

D.11 12.5 ml

D.12 2.5 ml

D.13 1 in 200,000 means 1 g in 200,000 ml. However, you have a 20 ml vial.

First convert 1 g to milligrams:

1,000 mg in 200,000 ml

Next work out how many mg in 1 ml:

$$1 \, \text{ml} = \frac{1,000}{200,000} \, \text{mg}$$

(using the '**one** unit' rule).

Now work out how much is in the 20 ml vial:

$$20\,\text{ml} = \frac{1,000}{200,000} \times 20 = 0.1\,\text{mg}$$

Answer: There are 0.1 mg or 100 mcg of adrenaline in a 20 ml vial containing 1 in 200,000.

D.14 1 in 100 means 1 g in 100 ml
1 g in 100 ml is equal to 1%

D.15 In this case the dose = 27,000 units. Therefore you would use:

$1 \times 25,000$ units/ml, 1 ml ampoule *plus*
$1 \times 5,000$ units/ml, 1 ml ampoule

Calculate how much of the 5,000 units/ml ampoule you need:

27,000 units − 25,000 units = 2,000 units

Therefore you need to draw up 2,000 units from the 5,000 units/ml ampoule.

Write down what you have, i.e. 5,000 units in 1 ml.
Work out the volume for 1 unit:

5,000 units in 1 ml

$$1\,\text{unit} = \frac{1}{5,000}\,\text{ml}$$

(using the '**one** unit' rule).

Now multiply by the dose required (2,000 units):

$$2,000\,\text{units} = \frac{1}{5,000} \times 2,000 = 0.4\,\text{ml}$$

Answer: You would add $1 \times 25,000$ units/ml ampoule and 0.4 ml of $1 \times 5,000$ units/ml to the infusion.

Alternatively, use the formula:

$$\frac{\text{Amount you want}}{\text{Amount you've got}} \times \text{Volume it's in}$$

Once again, before substituting numbers in the formula, decide as to which ampoule(s) of heparin would be the most appropriate; then, if necessary, calculate how much to draw up. Thus:

> Amount you want   = 2,000 units
> Amount you've got = 5,000 units
> Volume it's in   = 1 ml

Substitute the numbers in the formula:

$$\frac{2,000}{5,000} \times 1 = 0.4 \, \text{ml}$$

Answer: You would add 1 × 25,000 units/ml ampoule and 0.4 ml of 1 × 5,000 units/ml to the infusion.

D.16 Add 1 × 25,000 units/ml ampoule and 0.8 ml of 1 × 5,000 units/ml to the infusion

7 Preparation of solutions (dilutions)

INTRODUCTION

Most solutions are stored in a concentrated form in order to save storage space. The concentrated or stock solution is then diluted before use. The same stock solution may be used at different concentrations or strengths for different purposes.

The strengths of solutions, stock or diluted, may be stated in grams/litre, as ratio strengths (e.g. 1 in 10,000), or as percentage strengths.

It is unlikely that you will need to dilute solutions as these will be prepared in the pharmacy and sent to the ward ready for use.

However, you may need to prepare solutions for topical use, e.g. potassium permanganate; or perform simple dilutions, e.g. prepare half or quarter strength solutions.

PREPARATION OF SIMPLE SOLUTIONS

As stated before, it may be necessary to prepare solutions of various strengths from a stock solution.

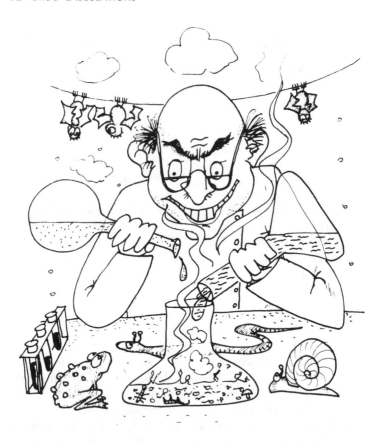

The principles are the same as in earlier calculations we've covered.

In this case, it is simply the dilution of a stock solution to the concentration or strength required by a diluent. The diluent is usually water, but occasionally other diluents are used.

The concentration required is usually written as a percentage (%v/v), i.e. the number of ml per 100 ml. Thus 45% v/v equals 45 ml per 100 ml.

For a fuller explanation of concentrations, see Section 6 on Drug strengths or concentrations.

WORKED EXAMPLE
Preparation of a solution from a stock solution

You need to prepare 500 ml of a 45% solution. What volume of stock solution do you need which when diluted to 500 ml will give a 45% solution?

In this case, the original volume of the stock solution does not matter. You are only interested in the final (diluted) solution and how much of the stock solution is needed to make the final solution.

Step 1
Convert the percentage required to the number of ml per 100 ml, i.e.

45% v/v = 45 ml in 100 ml

Thus for every 100 ml of your final solution, 45 ml will be the original or stock solution.

Step 2
Work out how much of the stock solution is needed for every 1 ml of the final solution, i.e. divide by 100:

45 ml in 100 ml

$$1 \text{ ml in } \frac{45}{100} \text{ ml}$$

(you are using the '**one** unit' rule).

Step 3
However, you need to prepare 500 ml for your final solution. Calculate the volume of stock solution required by multiplying the volume for 1 ml by the final volume, i.e.

$$1 \text{ ml in } \frac{45}{100} \text{ ml}$$

Thus for 500 ml, you will need:

$$\frac{45}{100} \times 500 = 225 \text{ ml}$$

Step 4

From step 3, you have just worked out that you need 225 ml of stock solution. Therefore you will need:

500 ml − 225 ml = 275 ml of diluent

Answer: To prepare 500 ml of a 45% solution, you will need 225 ml of stock solution diluted with 275 ml of diluent.

Alternatively, a simple formula can be used:

$$\text{Amount of stock solution required (in ml)} = \frac{\text{\% Concentration of the final solution}}{100} \times \text{Final volume required (in ml)}$$

where, in this example:

% Concentration of the final solution = 45%
Final volume required (in ml)　　　 = 500 ml

Substitute the figures in the formula:

$$\frac{45}{100} \times 500 = 225 \text{ ml}$$

Answer: To prepare 500 ml of a 45% solution, you will need 225 ml of stock solution diluted with 275 ml of diluent.

WORKED EXAMPLE
Preparation of a solution from a stock solution of a stated strength

You need to prepare 1 litre of a 20% solution from an 80% stock solution. How much stock solution do you need which when diluted to 1 litre will give a 20% solution?

In this example, you have to take into account the strength of the stock solution.

To be easier to understand, it is best to work in units of concentration, i.e. 20% = 20 units per 100 ml.

Step 1

Convert the percentage required to the number of units per 100 ml:

20% = 20 units per 100 ml

Step 2

Calculate how many units there are in 1 ml, i.e. divide by 100:

$$\frac{20}{100} \text{ units per 1 ml}$$

(you are using the '**one** unit' rule).

Step 3

Calculate the total number of units required by multiplying the number of units in 1 ml by the final volume, i.e.

$$\frac{20}{100} \times 1{,}000 = 200 \text{ units}$$

Thus in the final solution of 1 litre (1,000 ml), you will need a 'concentration' of 200 units.

Step 4

You have an 80% stock solution (80 units per 100 ml). For 1 litre of your final solution, you have worked out that you will need 200 units. Therefore you now need to find out what volume of stock solution is equal to 200 units.

Step 5

For your stock solution, calculate the volume for one unit, i.e.

80 units in 100 ml

$$1 \text{ unit in } \frac{100}{80} \text{ ml}$$

(you are using the '**one** unit' rule).

Step 6

However, you require a final solution containing 200 units.

To calculate the volume of stock solution needed, multiply the volume for 1 unit of stock solution by the total number of units in the final solution (200 units), i.e.

$$\frac{100}{80} \times 200 = 250 \text{ ml}$$

Step 7

From step 6, you have just worked out that you need 250 ml of stock solution. Therefore you will need:

1,000 ml − 250 ml = 750 ml of diluent

Answer: To prepare 1 litre of a 20% solution, you will need 250 ml of stock solution diluted with 750 ml of diluent.

Alternatively, a simple formula can be used:

$$\text{Amount of stock solution required (in ml)} = \frac{\% \text{ Concentration of the final solution}}{\% \text{ Concentration of the stock solution}} \times \text{Final volume required (in ml)}$$

where, in the example:

% Concentration of the final solution = 20%
% Concentration of the stock solution = 80%
Final volume required (in ml)   = 1,000 ml

Substitute the figures in the formula:

$$\frac{20}{80} \times 1,000 = 250 \text{ ml}$$

Answer: To prepare 1,000 ml of a 20% solution, you will need 250 ml of stock solution diluted with 750 ml of diluent.

PREPARATION OF SIMPLE SOLUTIONS (DILUTIONS) – SUMMARY

Simple dilutions:

$$\text{Amount of stock solution required (in ml)} = \frac{\% \text{ Concentration of the final solution}}{100} \times \text{Final volume required (in ml)}$$

Dilution of a stock solution of a stated strength:

$$\text{Amount of stock solution required (in ml)} = \frac{\text{\% Concentration of the final solution}}{\text{\% Concentration of the stock solution}} \times \text{Final volume required (in ml)}$$

PROBLEMS

E.1 What volume of stock solution is required to give 10 ml of a 90% solution?

E.2 What volume of stock solution is required to give 500 ml of a 20% solution?

E.3 What volume of stock solution is required for 1 litre of a 5% formalin solution?

E.4 What volume of stock solution is required to give 500 ml of a 45% solution from a 60% stock solution?

E.5 What volume of stock solution is required to give 50 ml of a 60% solution from an 80% stock solution?

E.6 (a) What volume of stock solution is required to give 200 ml of an 80% solution?

   (b) From that 80% solution you have just prepared, you now need to make three 100 ml solutions of 50%, 40% and 30%. For each strength, how much of the 80% solution do you need?

   (c) How much of the 80% solution do you have left?

PREPARATION OF SOLUTIONS FOR TOPICAL APPLICATION OR SOAKS

Although solutions for topical application, soaks or disinfectants are not usually made on the ward now, it still may be necessary to prepare potassium permanganate solutions for soaks.

These solutions are made from strong or concentrated stock solutions which are diluted to form weaker solutions.

These diluted solutions are often expressed in ratio strengths, i.e. '1 in ...' concentrations for example:

   1 in 10,000
   1 in 500

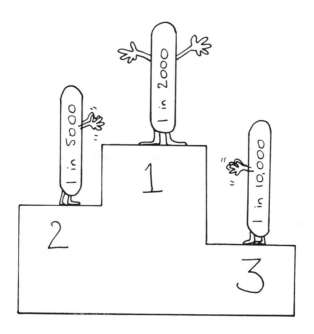

The 1 in 10,000 means 1 g dissolved in 10,000 ml. See Section 6 on Drug strengths or concentrations, for a fuller explanation.

Every ratio strength has an equivalent percentage strength and vice versa, and sometimes it is necessary to convert to a percentage (especially if you are using a formula). The following example shows you how this is done.

WORKED EXAMPLE

Convert a strength of 1 in 2,000 to a percentage.

Step 1
Write down what 1 in 2,000 means, i.e. 1 g in 2,000 ml.

Step 2
Calculate the number of grams in 1 ml, i.e. divide by 2,000:

$$\frac{1}{2,000} \text{ g in 1 ml}$$

(you are using the '**one** unit' rule).

Step 3
Percentage (%) means the number of grams per 100 ml. You
know the number of grams in 1 ml (step 2), thus to find how
many in 100 ml, multiply by 100:

$$\frac{1}{2,000} \times 100 = 0.05 \text{ g in 100 ml } (0.05\%)$$

So you are converting to a percentage.

Answer: 1 in 2,000 is equal to 0.05%.

A simple formula can be used to convert solution strengths to
percentages:

$$\text{Percentage} = \frac{1}{\text{Strength}} \times 100$$

Thus in the above example:

$$\text{Percentage} = \frac{1}{2,000} \times 100 = 0.05\%$$

Answer: 1 in 2,000 is equal to 0.05%.

PROBLEMS

Convert the following strengths to percentages:

E.7 1 in 800
E.8 1 in 20
E.9 1 in 4
E.10 1 in 20,000
E.11 1 in 500
E.12 1 in 5

WORKED EXAMPLE

Preparation of soaks

You need to prepare a potassium permanganate soak of 1 in 10,000. You have a stock solution of 10 g/litre. How much of the stock solution do you need to make a litre of a 1 in 10,000 solution?

When you are trying to solve these types of problems, it is much easier to work backwards and convert everything to the number of grams.

Step 1
Write down the final concentration required:

1 g in 10,000 ml (1 in 10,000)

Step 2
Next calculate how many grams (g) in 1 ml of your final solution by dividing by 10,000, i.e.

$$1\ \text{ml} = \frac{1}{10,000}\ \text{g}$$

Step 3
Now calculate the total number of grams for the final volume required, i.e. multiply the amount for 1 ml by 1,000 (1 litre = 1,000 ml). Thus:

$$1\ \text{ml} = \frac{1}{10,000}\ \text{g}$$

$$1,000\ \text{ml} = \frac{1}{10,000} \times 1,000\ \text{g}$$

You are converting the strength required (1 in 10,000) to the total number of grams or quantity required.

After calculating the number of grams in your final solution, you now need to work out how much of your stock solution is equal to the number of grams needed.

Step 4
Of the stock solution, calculate the volume for 1 g, i.e.

10 g in 1 litre *or* 10 g in 1,000 ml

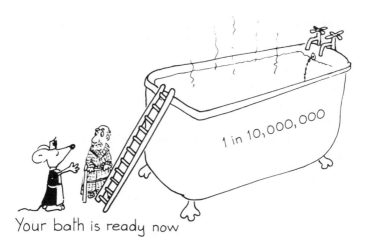

1 in 10,000,000

Your bath is ready now

Try to use practical units when performing dilutions

then

$$1\,g = \frac{1,000}{10}\,ml$$

Thus you are converting the strength of the stock solution to a volume containing 1 g.

Now calculate how much of the stock solution (in ml) is needed.

Step 5

To find out how much of the stock solution is needed, **multiply** the total number of grams in the final solution (step 3) by the volume for 1 g of stock solution (step 4), i.e.

$$\frac{1}{10,000} \times 1,000 \times \frac{1,000}{10} = \frac{100}{10} = 10\,ml$$

Therefore 10 ml of the stock solution is required.

Answer: 10 ml of a 10 g/litre stock solution when made up to 1 litre (1,000 ml) will give a 1 in 10,000 solution.

The same formula, as seen with the earlier dilution problems, can be used to work out the amount of stock solution needed:

$$\text{Amount of stock solution required (in ml)} = \frac{\text{Concentration of the final solution}}{\text{Concentration of the stock solution}} \times \text{Final volume required (in ml)}$$

The concentrations of the stock and final solutions can be expressed as either:

1. percentage concentration, or
2. a ratio strength (1 in ... concentration).

It is much easier to use percentage concentration, but both methods are being shown here using our original example.

WORKED EXAMPLE

1. Using percentage concentrations

The concentrations of the stock and final solutions must be converted to percentages:

$$\% \text{ Concentration of final solution} = \frac{1}{10,000} \times 100 = 0.01\%$$

$$\% \text{ Concentration of stock solution} = 10\,\text{g in }1,000\,\text{ml}$$
$$= 1\,\text{g in }100\,\text{ml} = 1\%$$

N.B. If the percentage concentration is not given for the stock solution, then it is assumed to be 100%.
Therefore you have:

% Concentration of the final solution = 0.01%
% Concentration of the stock solution = 1%
Final volume required (in ml)   = 1,000 ml

Substitute the figures in the formula:

$$\frac{0.01}{1} \times 1,000 = 10\,\text{ml}$$

Answer: 10 ml of the stock solution is required.

2. Using ratio strengths

If the stock solution is not given as a ratio strength, then you have to convert to a ratio strength.

In this case the stock solution = 10 g/litre or 10 g/1,000 ml.

This is equal to 1 g in 100 ml or, if written as a ratio strength, 1 in 100. (Ratio strengths are always '1 in . .' or '1 g in . . .'.)

However, if the stock solution is given as a percentage, convert to a fraction and then a ratio strength:

$$\frac{100}{\text{Percentage}} \text{ written as a '1 in . . .' answer}$$

In this case, the percentage of the stock solution = 1%, which is equal to:

$$\frac{100}{1} = 100, \text{ i.e. 1 in 100}$$

Therefore you have:

Concentration of the final solution = 1 in 10,000
Concentration of the stock solution = 1 in 100
Final volume required (in ml) = 1,000 ml

Substitute the figures in the formula:

$$\frac{1 \text{ in } 10,000}{1 \text{ in } 100} \times 1,000$$

This has to be rewritten as:

$$\frac{\dfrac{1}{10,000}}{\dfrac{1}{100}} \times 1,000$$

You always invert fractions when dividing, so this is equal to:

$$\frac{1}{10,000} \times \frac{100}{1} \times 1,000 = 10 \text{ ml}$$

Answer: 10 ml of the stock solution is required.

As you can see, using the formula can appear a bit complicated. However, if you work slowly and step by step, then you shouldn't have any problems.

Of the two methods, using percentage concentrations is the easier, but it is best to work from first principles.

If you are using the formula, take care with your calculations.

PREPARATION OF TOPICAL APPLICATIONS OR SOAKS – SUMMARY

Conversion of strengths to percentages:

$$\text{Percentage} = \frac{1}{\text{Strength}} \times 100$$

Preparation of soaks:

$$\text{Amount of stock solution required (in ml)} = \frac{\text{Concentration of the final solution}}{\text{Concentration of the stock solution}} \times \text{Final volume required (in ml)}$$

where the concentrations of the final and stock solutions are given as either **percentage concentrations** or **ratio strengths**.

PROBLEMS

E.13 You need to prepare a 1 in 15,000 solution of potassium permanganate. You have a stock solution of 10 g/litre and you will need a final volume of 3 litres. How much of the stock solution do you need which when diluted to 3 litres will give a 1 in 15,000 solution?

E.14 You need to prepare a litre of a 1 in 2,000 solution of chlorhexidine gluconate. You have a stock solution of 5%. How much of the stock solution do you need which when diluted to 1 litre will give a 1 in 2,000 solution?

E.15 You need to prepare a 1 in 10,000 solution of potassium permanganate. You have a stock solution of 10% and you will need a final volume of 1 litre. How much of the stock solution do you need which when diluted to 1 litre will give a 1 in 10,000 solution?

E.16 You need to prepare 500 ml of a 1 in 20 dilution of chloroxylenol. What volume of chloroxylenol do you need which when diluted to 500 ml will give a 1 in 20 dilution?

E.17 You need to prepare a litre of a 1 in 50,000 solution of potassium permanganate. You have a stock solution of 1 in 10,000 potassium permanganate. How much of the stock solution do you need which when diluted to 1 litre will give a 1 in 50,000 solution?

E.18 You need to prepare 500 ml of a 1 in 10,000 solution of potassium permanganate. You have a stock solution of 1 in 2,000 potassium permanganate. How much of the stock solution do you need which when diluted to 500 ml will give a 1 in 10,000 solution?

ANSWERS TO PROBLEMS

E.1 Convert the percentage required to the number of ml per 100 ml:

$$90\% = 90\,\text{ml in } 100\,\text{ml}$$

(Thus for every 100 ml of the final solution, 90 ml will be the stock solution.)

Now work out the volume of stock solution required for 1 ml of the final solution:

$$1\,\text{ml} = \frac{90}{100}\,\text{ml}$$

However, the final volume required is 10 ml, so

$$10\,\text{ml} = \frac{90}{100} \times 10 = 9\,\text{ml}$$

Answer: 9 ml of stock solution when diluted to 10 ml will give a 90% solution.

Or by using the formula:

$$\text{Amount of stock solution required (in ml)} = \frac{\text{\% Concentration of the final solution}}{100} \times \text{Final volume required (in ml)}$$

where in this case:

%️ Concentration of the final solution = 90%
Final volume required = 10 ml

substitute the figures in the formula:

$$\frac{90}{100} \times 10 = 9\,\text{ml}$$

Answer: 9 ml of stock solution when diluted to 10 ml will give a 90% solution.

E.2 100 ml
E.3 50 ml
E.4 375 ml
E.5 37.5 ml
E.6 (a) To prepare 200 ml of an 80% solution, convert the percentage required to the number of ml per 100 ml:

80% = 80 ml per 100 ml

Work out how many ml of stock solution there are in 1 ml of the final solution, i.e. divide by 100:

$$\frac{80}{100} = 0.8\,\text{ml}$$

To find out how much stock solution you need, multiply by the final volume (200 ml):

$$0.8 \times 200 = 160\,\text{ml}$$

Or by using the formula:

$$\text{Amount of stock solution required (in ml)} = \frac{\text{\% Concentration of the final solution}}{100} \times \text{Final volume required (in ml)}$$

where in this case:

% Concentration of the final solution = 80%
Final volume required   = 200 ml

substitute the figures in the formula:

$$\frac{80}{100} \times 200 = 160 \, ml$$

(b) You now have 200 ml of an 80% solution. To prepare 100 ml of a 50% solution, convert the percentage required to the number of units per 100 ml:

50% = 50 units per 100 ml

Calculate how many units there are in 1 ml, i.e. divide by 100:

$$\frac{50}{100} \, units \, per \, ml$$

Calculate the total number of units required by multiplying by the final volume (100 ml):

$$\frac{50}{100} \times 100 = 50 \, units$$

However, you have a stock solution of 80%:

80% = 80 units per 100 ml

This time, calculate the number of ml for 1 unit of stock solution, i.e. divide by 100:

$$1 \, unit = \frac{100}{80} \, ml$$

Calculate the volume of stock solution required by multiplying the volume for 1 unit of stock solution by the total number of units required to make your solution:

$$\frac{100}{80} \times 50 = 62.5 \, ml$$

Consequently:

For 40%, you will need 50 ml of the 80% solution
For 30%, you will need 37.5 ml of the 80% solution

Or by using the formula:

$$\begin{array}{l} \text{Amount of stock} \\ \text{solution required} \\ \text{(in ml)} \end{array} = \dfrac{\begin{array}{c}\text{\% Concentration of}\\\text{the final solution}\end{array}}{\begin{array}{c}\text{\% Concentration of}\\\text{the stock solution}\end{array}} \times \begin{array}{l}\text{Final volume}\\\text{required}\\\text{(in ml)}\end{array}$$

where in this example:

% Concentration of the final solution = 50%
% Concentration of the stock solution = 80%
Final volume required (in ml)   = 100 ml

substitute the figures in the formula:

$$\frac{50}{80} \times 100 = 62.5\,\text{ml}$$

Consequently:

For 40%, you will need 50 ml of the 80% solution
For 30%, you will need 37.5 ml of the 80% solution

(c) Total volume required equals

62.5 ml + 50 ml + 37.5 ml = 150 ml

Amount left will therefore be 200 ml − 150 ml = 50 ml.

E.7 0.125%

E.8 5%

E.9 25%

E.10 0.005% (5×10^{-3})

E.11 0.2%

E.12 20%

E.13 Write down the final concentration required:

1 in 15,000 equals 1 g in 15,000 ml

Now work out the number of grams in 1 ml of the final solution:

$$1\,\text{ml} = \frac{1}{15,000}\,\text{g}$$

Next work out the number of grams in the final volume, 3 litres (3,000 ml):

$$3,000\,\text{ml} = \frac{1}{15,000} \times 3,000\,\text{g}$$

Now work out how much stock solution is required. First, calculate the volume (in ml) for 1 g of stock solution. You have:

10 g in 1 litre or 10 g in 1,000 ml

Therefore

$$1\,g = \frac{10,000}{10}\,ml$$

Second, multiply the number of grams in the final solution by the volume of stock solution for 1 g, i.e.

$$\frac{1}{15,000} \times 3,000 \times \frac{1,000}{10} = \frac{300}{15} = 20\,ml$$

Answer: 20 ml of the stock solution is required.

Or by using the formula:

$$\begin{array}{c} \text{Amount of stock} \\ \text{solution required} \\ \text{(in ml)} \end{array} = \dfrac{\begin{array}{c}\% \text{ Concentration of} \\ \text{the final solution}\end{array}}{\begin{array}{c}\% \text{ Concentration of} \\ \text{the stock solution}\end{array}} \times \begin{array}{c} \text{Final volume} \\ \text{required} \\ \text{(in ml)} \end{array}$$

where in this case:

$$\% \text{ Concentration of final solution} = \frac{1}{15,000} \times 100$$
$$= 0.0067\%$$
% Concentration of stock solution = 10 g in 1,000 ml
$$= 1\,g \text{ in } 100\,ml = 1\%$$
Final volume required = 3,000 ml (3 litres)

substitute the figures in the formula:

$$\frac{0.0067}{1} \times 3,000 = 20.1\,ml$$

Answer: 20 ml of the stock solution is required.

E.14 10 ml

E.15 1 ml

E.16 25 ml (assume the chloroxylenol = 100%)

E.17 200 ml

E.18 100 ml

8 *Moles and millimoles*

INTRODUCTION

Daily references may be made to moles and millimoles in relation to 'electrolyte levels', 'blood glucose', 'serum creatinine', or other blood results with regard to patients. These terms refer to measurements carried out by biochemists in chemical pathology to determine the amounts of particular substances in the body fluids of the patient. They are also used when adding electrolytes to infusions, e.g. potassium chloride. These measurements are usually expressed in **millimoles**. For example:

Mr. J. Brown   Sodium = 138 mmol/L

Add 20 mmol potassium chloride to an infusion

Before you can interpret such results or amounts, you will need to be familiar with this rather confusing unit: the **mole**.

The following will try and explain what moles and millimoles are, and how to do calculations involving millimoles.

WHAT ARE MOLES AND MILLIMOLES?

The concept of moles and millimoles is difficult to understand, but it is important to know what moles and millimoles are and how they are derived. First you need to be familiar with some basic chemistry: atoms and molecules.

Counting atoms

Relative atomic masses show that one atom of carbon is 12 times as heavy as one atom of hydrogen. Therefore, 12 g of carbon will contain the same number of atoms as 1 g of hydrogen.

In fact, *the relative atomic mass (in grams) of every element* (1 g of hydrogen, 12 g carbon, 16 g oxygen, etc.) *will contain the same number of atoms*. This number is called **Avogadro's constant** in honour of the Italian scientist Amedeo Avogadro. *The relative atomic mass is known as* **one mole** *of the element*. So 12 g of carbon and 1 g of hydrogen is also one mole. 24 g of carbon is 2 moles and 36 g of carbon is 3 moles, etc.

Experiments show that Avogadro's constant is equal to 6×10^{23}. When this notation is written out in full, it is equal to 600,000,000,000,000,000,000,000, showing that it is a very large number! Thus 1 mole of an element will always contain 6×10^{23} atoms.

This counting of atoms or moles is used to measure the 'amount' of a substance:

12 g of carbon = 1 mole or 6×10^{23} atoms
1 g of carbon = $\frac{1}{12}$ mole or $\frac{1}{12} \times 6 \times 10^{23}$ atoms
10 g of carbon = $\frac{10}{12}$ mole or $\frac{10}{12} \times 6 \times 10^{23}$ atoms

Chemists are not the only people who 'count by weighing'. Bank clerks use the same idea when they count coins by weighing them. For example, 100 1p coins weigh 356 g; so it is quicker to weigh 356 g of 1p coins than to count 100 coins.

To get the right quantities, chemists must measure in moles and *not* in grams. Thus the mole is the chemist's counting unit.

So how can we relate this to everyday units?

As stated before, the mole is the S.I. unit for the amount of substance.

TABLE 8.1 Atomic and molecular masses

Calcium (Ca)	= 40
Calcium chloride	= 147
Calcium gluconate	= 448.5
Carbon (C)	= 12
Chloride (Cl)	= 35.5
Dextrose/Glucose	= 180
Hydrogen (H)	= 1
Lactic acid	= 90
Magnesium (Mg)	= 24
Magnesium chloride	= 203
Magnesium sulphate	= 246.5
Oxygen (O)	= 16
Potassium (K)	= 39
Potassium chloride	= 74.5
Sodium (Na)	= 23
Sodium bicarbonate	= 84
Sodium chloride	= 58.5
Sodium phosphate	= 358

The reason why sometimes the molecular mass does not equal the sum of the atomic masses of the individual atoms is that water forms part of the molecule. For example, calcium chloride is *not* $CaCl_2$ but is actually $CaCl_2.2H_2O$.

The relative atomic mass for carbon = 12 (see Table 8.1). Since one mole is equal to 12 g of carbon, it follows that:

One mole = the **relative atomic mass** in grams

Now consider molecules:

Sodium chloride (NaCl)

Sodium chloride is made up of two atoms or ions: sodium (Na) and chloride (Cl):

$$Na \quad Cl \qquad = molecule$$

$$Na^+ \qquad Cl^- \qquad = ions$$

The individual parts of the molecule are called ions. Thus in the above example, NaCl (sodium chloride) is the molecule, and the Na^+ (sodium) and Cl^- (chloride) are the ions.

Hence 1 mole of sodium chloride provides or gives 1 mole of sodium ions and 1 mole of chloride ions.

From Table 8.1 the relative atomic masses of:

Sodium (Na)   = 23
Chloride (Cl) = 35.5

The molecular mass is the sum of the relative atomic masses, i.e. in this case:

Sodium (Na)   = 23
Chloride (Cl) $= \dfrac{35.5}{58.5}$ = molecular mass

Thus in this case:

One mole = the **molecular mass** in grams

The quantity of the molecules (in grams) containing 1 mole of a particular ion or atom can be found by dividing the molecular mass by the number of that ion or atom contained in the molecule.

Sodium chloride (NaCl), molecular mass = 58.5 g, contains one ion of sodium (Na) and one ion of chloride (Cl).

Thus to obtain 1 mole of sodium ions, you will need 1 mole of sodium chloride.

So the amount needed (in grams) for 1 mole of sodium is given by:

$$\frac{\text{Molecular mass}}{\text{Number of ions}} = \frac{58.5}{1} = 58.5$$

Thus 58.5 g of sodium chloride will give 1 mole of sodium ions.

Now consider carbon dioxide (CO_2). It consists of one carbon atom and two oxygen atoms. The '2' after the 'O' means two atoms of oxygen:

C O_2 = molecule

C   O + O   = atoms

The individual parts of the molecule are called atoms. Thus in the above example, CO_2 (carbon dioxide) is the molecule, and the C (carbon) and O (oxygen) are the atoms.

Hence 1 mole of carbon dioxide provides or gives 1 mole of carbon atoms and 2 moles of oxygen atoms.

From Table 8.1 the relative atomic masses of:

Carbon (C) = 12
Oxygen (O) = 16

The molecular mass is the sum of the relative atomic masses, i.e. in this case:

Carbon (C)   = 12

Oxygen (O) = 2 × 16 = 32

                                            44 = molecular mass

Thus in this case:

One mole = the molecular mass in grams

The quantity of the molecules (in grams) containing 1 mole of a particular ion or atom can be found by dividing the molecular mass by the number of that ion or atom contained in the molecule.

Carbon dioxide (CO_2), molecular mass = 44 g, contains one atom of carbon (C) and two atoms of oxygen (O).

Thus to obtain 1 mole of carbon atoms, you will need 1 mole of carbon dioxide.

So the amount needed (in grams) for 1 mole of carbon is given by:

$$\frac{\text{Molecular mass}}{\text{Number of atoms}} = \frac{44}{1} = 44$$

Thus 44 g of carbon dioxide will give 1 mole of carbon atoms.

However, to obtain 1 mole of oxygen atoms, you will need $\frac{1}{2}$ mole of carbon dioxide (1 mole of carbon dioxide contains 2 moles of oxygen).

So the amount needed (in grams) for 1 mole of oxygen is given by:

$$\frac{\text{Molecular mass}}{\text{Number of atoms}} = \frac{44}{2} = 22$$

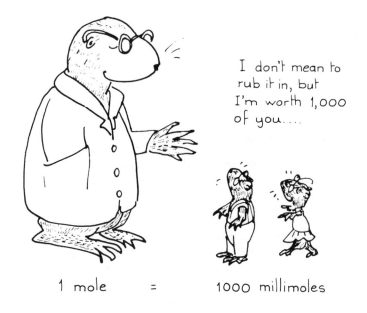

I don't mean to
rub it in, but
I'm worth 1,000
of you....

1 mole = 1000 millimoles

Thus 22 g of carbon dioxide will give 1 mole of oxygen atoms.

The millimole

In practice, moles are too big for everyday use, so **millimoles** are used. One millimole is equal to $\frac{1}{1,000}$ of a mole.

One mole is the atomic mass or molecular mass in grams. Therefore one millimole is the atomic mass or molecular mass in milligrams.

So, in the above explanation, you can substitute millimoles for moles and milligrams for grams.

The following worked examples and problems will help you to understand the concept of millimoles. It is unlikely that you will encounter these types of calculations on the ward, but it is useful to know how they are done and this section can be used for reference if necessary.

CONVERSION OF MILLIGRAMS (mg) TO MILLIMOLES (mmol)

Sometimes it may be necessary to calculate the number of millimoles in an infusion or injection or to convert mg/litre to mmol/litre.

WORKED EXAMPLE

How many millimoles of sodium are there in a 500 ml infusion containing 1.8 mg/ml sodium chloride?

Step 1
As already stated, one millimole of sodium chloride yields one millimole of sodium and one millimole of chloride.

So it follows that the amount (in milligrams) equal to one millimole of sodium chloride will give one millimole of sodium.

In this case, calculate the total amount (in milligrams) of sodium chloride and convert this to millimoles to find out the number of millimoles of sodium.

Step 2
Calculate the total amount of sodium chloride. You have an infusion containing 1.8 mg/ml. Therefore in 500 ml, you have:

$$1.8 \times 500 = 900 \text{ mg sodium chloride}$$

Step 3
From Table 8.1, molecular mass of sodium chloride (NaCl) = 58.5. So one millimole of sodium chloride (NaCl) will weigh 58.5 mg and this amount will give one millimole of sodium (Na).

Step 4
Next calculate the number of millimoles in the infusion. First work out the number of millimoles for 1 mg of sodium chloride, then the number for the total amount. 58.5 mg sodium chloride will give 1 millimole of sodium. Therefore 1 mg will give:

$\dfrac{1}{58.5}$ millimoles of sodium

So, 900 mg will give

$\dfrac{1}{58.5} \times 900 = 15.4$ mmol (or 15 mmol approx.)

Answer: There are 15.4 mmol (approximately 15 mmol) of sodium in a 500 ml infusion containing 1.8 mg/ml sodium chloride.

Alternatively, a formula can be used:

$$\text{Total number} = \dfrac{\text{mg/ml}}{\substack{\text{mg of substance} \\ \text{containing 1 mmol}}} \times \text{Volume (in ml)}$$

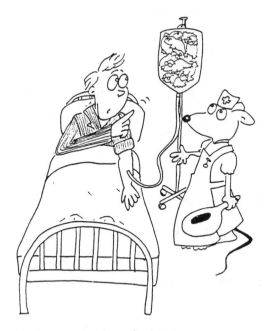

Well, yes…. the drug chart <u>did</u> say
100 millimoles/litre but I could
only squeeze in 10!

where in this case:

```
mg/ml                                = 1.8 mg/ml
mg of substance containing 1 mmol = 58.5 mg
Volume                               = 500 ml
```

Substitute the numbers in the formula:

$$\frac{1.8}{58.5} \times 500 = 15.38 \text{ mmol (or 15 mmol approx.)}$$

Answer: There are 15.4 mmol (approximately 15 mmol) of sodium in a 500 ml infusion containing 1.8 mg/ml sodium chloride.

However, if you are given the total amount in mg/litre, the calculations are the same. In this example, the total amount per litre would be 1,800 mg/litre.

WORKED EXAMPLE

How many millimoles of sodium are there in a 1 litre infusion containing 1,800 mg/litre sodium chloride?

58.5 mg sodium chloride will give 1 millimole of sodium. Therefore 1 mg will give:

$$\frac{1}{58.5} \text{ millimoles of sodium}$$

So, 1,800 mg will give:

$$\frac{1}{58.5} \times 1,800 = 30.8 \text{ mmol (or 31 mmol approx.)}$$

Answer: An infusion containing 1,800 mg/litre of sodium chloride contains 31 mmol/litre of sodium (approx.).

The formula can be rewritten as:

$$\text{mmol/litre} = \frac{\text{mg/litre}}{\text{mg of substance containing 1 mmol}}$$

where in this case:

mg/litre   = 1,800 mg/litre
mg of substance containing 1 mmol = 58.5 mg

Substitute the numbers in the formula:

$$\frac{1,800}{58.5} = 30.8 \text{ mmol (or 31 mmol approx.)}$$

Answer: An infusion containing 1,800 mg/litre of sodium chloride contains 31 mmol/litre of sodium (approx.).

MOLES AND MILLIMOLES 1 – SUMMARY

One mole (mol) is the atomic or molecular mass in grams

One millimole (mmol) is the atomic or molecular mass in milligrams

N.B. 1 millimole is one-thousandth of a mole, i.e.

$$1 \text{ mmol} = \frac{1}{1,000} \text{ mol}$$

Conversion of mg/ml to millimoles (mmol):

$$\text{Total number of millimoles} = \frac{\text{mg/ml}}{\text{mg of substance containing 1 mmol}} \times \text{Volume (in ml)}$$

Conversion of mg/litre to mmol/litre:

$$\text{mmol/litre} = \frac{\text{mg/litre}}{\text{mg of substance containing 1 mmol}}$$

PROBLEMS

F.1 How many millimoles of sodium are there in a 500 ml infusion containing 27 mg/ml sodium chloride?

F.2 How many millimoles of sodium are there in a 10 ml ampoule containing 200 mg/ml sodium chloride?

F.3 How many millimoles of sodium, potassium and chloride are there in a 500 ml infusion containing 9 mg/ml sodium chloride and 3 mg/ml potassium chloride?

F.4 How many millimoles of glucose are there in a litre infusion containing 50 g/litre?

F.5 How many millimoles of sodium are there in a litre infusion containing 27.4 g/litre sodium bicarbonate?

F.6 You need to draw up 35 mmol of potassium chloride and to add this to a litre infusion. You have an ampoule containing 2 g of potassium chloride in 10 ml. How much do you need to draw up?

F.7 You need to draw up 15 mmol of potassium chloride and to add this to a litre infusion. You have an ampoule containing 1 g of potassium chloride in 5 ml. How much do you need to draw up?

CONVERSION OF PERCENTAGE STRENGTH (% w/v) TO MILLIMOLES

It may be necessary to convert percentages to the number of millimoles.

WORKED EXAMPLE

How many millimoles of sodium are in 1 litre of sodium chloride 0.9% infusion?

Step 1

As before, one millimole of sodium chloride will give one millimole of sodium and one millimole of chloride.

So, the amount (in milligrams) equal to one millimole of sodium chloride will give one millimole of sodium.

Step 2

To calculate the number of milligrams there are in one millimole of sodium chloride, either refer to Table 8.1 or work from first principles using atomic masses.

From Table 8.1, molecular mass of sodium chloride (NaCl) = 58.5. So one millimole of sodium chloride (NaCl) will weigh 58.5 mg and this amount will give one millimole of sodium (Na).

Step 3

Calculate the total amount of sodium chloride present:

$$0.9\% = 0.9\,g \text{ in } 100\,ml$$
$$= 900\,mg \text{ in } 100\,ml$$

Thus for a 1 litre (1,000 ml) infusion bag, the amount equals:

$$\frac{900}{100} \times 1,000 = 9,000\,mg \text{ or } 9\,g$$

Step 4

From step 2, it was found that 58.5 mg sodium chloride will give one millimole of sodium. So it follows that 1 mg of sodium chloride will give:

$$\frac{1}{58.5} \text{ millimoles of sodium}$$

So 9,000 mg sodium chloride will give:

$$\frac{1}{58.5} \times 9,000 = 153.8 \text{ (154) mmol of sodium}$$

Answer: 1 litre of sodium chloride 0.9% infusion contains 154 mmol of sodium (approx.).

A formula can be devised:

$$\frac{\text{Total number}}{\text{of mmol}} = \frac{\text{Percentage strength (\% w/v)}}{\text{mg of substance containing 1 mmol}}$$
$$\times 10 \times \text{Volume (ml)}$$

where in this case:

Percentage strength (% w/v)   = 0.9%
mg of substance containing 1 mmol = 58.5 mg
Volume   = 1,000 ml

The '10' simply converts percentage strength (g/100 ml) to mg/ml (everything in the same units).

Substituting the numbers in the formula:

$$\frac{0.9}{58.5} \times 10 \times 1,000 = 153.8 \ (154) \ \text{mmol of sodium}$$

Answer: 1 litre of sodium chloride 0.9% infusion contains 154 mmol of sodium (approx.).

MOLES AND MILLIMOLES 2 – SUMMARY

Conversion of percentage strength (% w/v) to millimoles (mmol):

$$\text{Total number of millimoles} = \frac{\text{Percentage strength (\% w/v)}}{\text{mg of substance containing 1 mmol}} \times 10 \times \text{Volume (ml)}$$

PROBLEMS

F.8 How many millimoles of sodium are there in a 1 litre infusion of glucose 4% and sodium chloride 0.18%?

F.9 How many millimoles of calcium and chloride are there in a 10 ml ampoule of calcium chloride 10%? N.B. Calcium chloride = $CaCl_2$

F.10 How many millimoles of sodium are there in a 10 ml ampoule of sodium chloride 30%?

F.11 How many millimoles of calcium are there in a 10 ml ampoule of calcium gluconate 10%?

F.12 How many millimoles of sodium are there in a 200 ml infusion of sodium bicarbonate 8.4%?

ANSWERS TO PROBLEMS

F.1 One millimole of sodium chloride will give one millimole of sodium and one millimole of chloride. So the amount (in milligrams) for one millimole of sodium chloride will give one millimole of sodium.

From Table 8.1, the molecular mass of sodium chloride = 58.5.

So 58.5 mg (one millimole) of sodium chloride will give one millimole of sodium.

Thus it follows that 1 mg of sodium chloride will give

$$\frac{1}{58.5} \text{ millimoles of sodium}$$

Now work out the total amount of sodium chloride in a 500 ml infusion. You have 27 mg/ml, thus for 500 ml:

$$27 \times 500 = 13,500 \text{ mg}$$

Next work out the number of millimoles for the infusion:

$$1 \text{ mg will give } \frac{1}{58.5} \text{ millimoles}$$

$$13,500 \text{ mg will give } \frac{1}{58.5} \times 13,500 = 230.8 \ (231) \text{ mmol}$$

Answer: There are 231 mmol (approx.) of sodium in a 500 ml infusion containing sodium chloride 27 mg/ml.

If using the formula:

$$\text{Total number of millimoles} = \frac{\text{mg/ml}}{\text{mg of substance containing 1 mmol}} \times \text{Volume (in ml)}$$

where in this case

mg/ml = 27 mg/ml
mg of substance containing 1 mmol = 58.5 mg
Volume = 500 ml

substitute the numbers in the formula:

$$\frac{27}{58.5} \times 500 = 230.8 \ (231) \ \text{mmol}$$

Answer: There are 231 mmol (approx.) of sodium in a 500 ml infusion containing sodium chloride 27 mg/ml.

F.2 34.2 mmol (34 mmol, approx.) of sodium

F.3 Sodium   76.9 mmol (77 mmol, approx.)
Potassium   20.2 mmol (20 mmol, approx.)
Chloride   97.2 mmol (97 mmol, approx.)

One millimole of potassium chloride gives one millimole of potassium and *one* millimole of chloride.

One millimole of sodium chloride gives one millimole of sodium and *one* millimole of chloride.

Thus to find the total amount of chloride, add the amount for the sodium and potassium together.

F.4 277.8 mmol (278 mmol, approx.) of glucose

F.5 326.2 mmol (326 mmol, approx.) of sodium

F.6 One millimole of potassium chloride gives one millimole of potassium and one millimole of chloride.

From Table 8.1, the molecular mass of potassium chloride = 74.5. Thus one millimole of potassium chloride = 74.5 mg. Therefore:

$$35 \ \text{mmol} = 74.5 \times 35 = 2{,}607.5 \ \text{mg}$$

To work out the volume required, you have 2 g (2,000 mg) in 10 ml; thus

$$1 \ \text{mg} = \frac{10}{2{,}000} \ \text{ml}$$

Therefore for 2,607.5 mg, you will need:

$$\frac{10}{2{,}000} \times 2{,}607.5 = 13.04 \ \text{ml}$$

Answer: You will need to draw up 13 ml.

Or use the formula:

$$\text{Total number of millimoles} = \frac{\text{mg/ml}}{\text{mg of substance containing 1 mmol}} \times \text{Volume (in ml)}$$

In this case, the unknown is the volume (the volume you need to draw up). So the formula can be rewritten as:

$$\text{Volume (in ml)} = \frac{\text{mg of substance containing 1 mmol}}{\text{mg/ml}} \times \text{Total number of millimoles}$$

where in this case:

mg of substance containing 1 mmol = 74.5 mg
mg/ml   = 200 mg/ml
Total number of millimoles   = 35 mmol

Substitute the numbers in the formula:

$$\frac{74.5}{200} \times 35 = 13.04 \ (13) \ \text{ml}$$

Answer: You will need to draw up 13 ml.

F.7 You will need to draw up 5.6 ml.

F.8 In this question, ignore the glucose since it contains no sodium; simply consider the infusion as sodium chloride 0.18%.

One millimole of sodium chloride will give one millimole of sodium and one millimole of chloride. So the amount (in milligrams) for one millimole of sodium chloride will give one millimole of sodium.

From Table 8.1, the molecular mass of sodium chloride = 58.5. So 58.5 mg (one millimole) of sodium chloride will give one millimole of sodium.

Now work out the number of millimoles for 1 mg of sodium chloride:

58.5 mg sodium chloride will give 1 millimole of sodium

1 mg sodium chloride will give $\frac{1}{58.5}$ millimoles of sodium

Next, calculate the total amount of sodium chloride present:

0.18% = 0.18 g or 180 mg per 100 ml

Therefore in 1 litre:

180 × 10 = 1,800 mg sodium chloride

Now calculate the number of millimoles for 1,800 mg sodium chloride:

$$1,800 \text{ mg} = \frac{1}{58.5} \times 1,800 = 30.8 \text{ (31) mmol}$$

Answer: 1 litre of glucose 4% and sodium chloride 0.18% infusion contains 31 mmol of sodium (approx.).

If using the formula:

$$\text{Total number} = \frac{\text{Percentage strength (\% w/v)}}{\substack{\text{mg of substance containing} \\ 1 \text{ mmol}}}$$

$$\times 10 \times \text{Volume (ml)}$$

where in this case:

Percentage strength (% w/v) $= 0.18\%$
mg of substance containing 1 mmol $= 58.5 \text{ mg}$
Volume $= 1,000 \text{ ml}$

substitute the numbers in the formula:

$$\frac{0.18}{58.5} \times 10 \times 1,000 = 30.8 \text{ (31) mmol of sodium}$$

Answer: 1 litre of glucose 4% and sodium chloride 0.9% infusion contains 31 mmol of sodium (approx.).

F.9 In this case one millimole of calcium chloride will give one millimole of calcium and *two* millimoles of chloride. So the amount (in milligrams) for one millimole of calcium chloride will give one millimole of calcium and *two* millimoles of chloride.

From Table 8.1, the molecular mass of calcium chloride = 147. So 147 mg (one millimole) of calcium chloride will give one millimole of calcium and two millimoles of chloride.

Now calculate how much calcium chloride there is in a 10 ml ampoule containing calcium chloride 10%.

10% = 10 g in 100 ml, therefore 1 g or 1,000 mg in 10 ml

Calcium
One millimole of calcium is equal to 147 mg of calcium
chloride. Therefore 1 mg calcium chloride is equal to

$$\frac{1}{147} \text{ mmol of calcium}$$

However, you have 1,000 mg of calcium chloride. Thus:

$$1,000 \text{ mg} = \frac{1}{147} \times 1,000 = 6.8 \text{ mmol (7 mmol, approx.)}$$

Chloride
Two millimoles of chloride is equal to 147 mg of calcium
chloride. Therefore 1 mg calcium chloride is equal to

$$\frac{2}{147} \text{ mmol of chloride}$$

However, you have 1,000 mg of calcium chloride. Thus:

$$1,000 \text{ mg} = \frac{2}{147} \times 1,000 = 13.6 \text{ mmol (14 mmol, approx.)}$$

Answer: There are 7 millimoles of calcium and 14 millimoles
of chloride in a 10 ml ampoule of calcium chloride 10%
(approx.).

Or use the formula:

$$\text{Total number} = \frac{\text{Percentage strength (\% w/v)}}{\text{mg of substance containing 1 mmol}}$$

$$\times 10 \times \text{Volume (ml)}$$

Calcium
In this case:

Percentage strength (% w/v)   = 10%
mg of substance containing 1 mmol = 147 mg
Volume   = 10 ml

Substitute the numbers in the formula:

$$\frac{10}{147} \times 10 \times 10 = 6.8 \text{ mmol (7 mmol, approx.)}$$

Chloride
In this case:

> Percentage strength (% w/v)   = 10%
> mg of substance containing 1 mmol = 73.5 mg
> Volume   = 10 ml

N.B. Mass (mg) of substance containing 1 mmol = 73.5 mg. This is because 2 mmol of chloride = 147 mg, thus 1 mmol chloride = 147/2 = 73.5 mg.

Substitute the numbers in the formula:

$$\frac{10}{73.5} \times 10 \times 10 = 13.6 \text{ mmol (14 mmol, approx.)}$$

Answer: There are 7 millimoles of calcium and 14 millimoles of chloride in a 10 ml ampoule of calcium chloride 10% (approx.).

F.10 51.28 mmol (51 mmol, approx.)
F.11 2.23 mmol (2 mmol, approx.)
F.12 200 mmol

9 *Intravenous therapy*

Infusion rate calculations

OBJECTIVES

At the end of this section you should be familiar with the following:

Giving sets

Calculating I.V. infusion rates (drops/min)

Conversion of infusion rates (ml/hour) to drops/min

Conversion of dosages to drops/min and ml/hour

Conversion of ml/hour to dosages

Calculating the length of time for I.V. infusions

Calculating infusion regimens

INTRODUCTION

Before doing any calculations, it is important to decide which **giving set** is going to be used as each giving set has a different drip rate.

Giving sets

There are two giving sets:

1. The **standard** giving set (SGS) has a drip rate of *20 drops per ml* for crystalloids (i.e. sodium chloride, dextrose) and *15 drops per ml* for colloids (e.g. blood).
2. The **microdrop** giving set or burette has a drip rate of *60 drops per ml*.

The drip rate of the giving set is always written on the wrapper if you are not sure.

Infusion rate calculations

In all infusion rate calculations, you have to remember that you are simply converting a volume to drops (or vice versa) and hours to minutes.

The following examples are hopefully the type of calculation you will encounter on the ward.

The principles learnt in this section can be applied to any calculation not dealt with here.

CALCULATING I.V. INFUSION RATES (drops/min)

When calculating infusion drip rates, it is necessary to decide which giving set you are going to use.

Usually a standard giving set (20 drops/ml) is used. A microdrop giving set or burette (60 drops/ml) is used when giving infusions very accurately.

WORKED EXAMPLE

1 litre of 5% dextrose is to be given over 8 hours. What drip rate is required?

You decide to use a standard giving set (SGS), 20 drops/ml.

Step 1
First convert the volume to a number of drops. To do this, multiply the volume of the infusion by the number of drops per ml for the giving set, i.e.

$1,000 \times 20 = 20,000$ drops

Thus for the giving set being used, you have just calculated the number of drops to be infused.

Step 2
Next convert hours to minutes by multiplying the number of hours for which the infusion is to be given by 60 (60 minutes = 1 hour):

8 hours = $8 \times 60 = 480$ minutes

Now everything has been converted in terms of drops and minutes, i.e. what you want for your final answer.

If the infusion is being given over a period of minutes, then obviously there is no need to convert from hours to minutes.

Step 3
Write down what you have just calculated, i.e. the total number of drops to be given over how many minutes.

20,000 drops to be given over 480 minutes

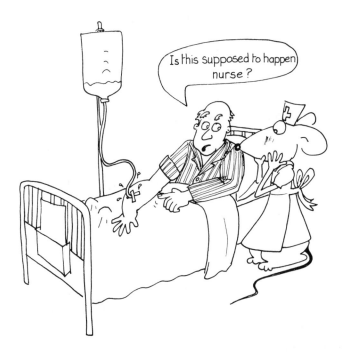

Step 4
Calculate the number of drops per minute by dividing the number of drops by the number of minutes, i.e.

20,000 drops over 480 minutes

$$\frac{20,000}{480} = 41.67 \text{ drops/min}$$

Since it is impossible to give part of a drop, round up or down to the nearest whole number:

41.67 = 42 drops/min

Answer: To give a litre (1,000 ml) of 5% dextrose over 8 hours, the rate will have to be 42 drops/min using a standard giving set (20 drops/ml).

A formula can be used:

$$\text{Drops/min} = \frac{\text{Drops/ml of the giving set} \times \text{Volume of the infusion}}{\text{Number of hours the infusion is to run} \times 60}$$

where in this case:

Drops/ml of the giving set = 20 drops/ml (SGS)
Volume of the infusion (in ml) = 1,000 ml
Number of hours the infusion is to run = 8 hours
60 = number of minutes in an hour (× 60 converts hours to minutes)

Substitute the numbers in the formula:

$$\frac{20 \times 1,000}{8 \times 60} = 41.67 \text{ drops/min (42 drops/min, approx.)}$$

Answer: To give a litre (1,000 ml) of 5% dextrose over 8 hours, the rate will have to be 42 drops/min using a standard giving set (20 drops/ml).

N.B. If the infusion is to run over a period of minutes instead of hours, then the formula will have to be rewritten:

$$\text{Drops/min} = \frac{\text{Drops/ml of the giving set} \times \text{Volume of the infusion}}{\text{Number of minutes the infusion is to run}}$$

CALCULATING INFUSION RATES
(drops/min) – SUMMARY

Infusion being given over a number of hours:

$$\text{Drops/min} = \frac{\text{Drops/ml of the giving set} \times \text{Volume of the infusion}}{\text{Number of hours the infusion is to run} \times 60}$$

Infusion being given over a number of minutes:

$$\text{Drops/min} = \frac{\text{Drops/ml of the giving set} \times \text{Volume of the infusion}}{\text{Number of minutes the infusion is to run}}$$

PROBLEMS

When answering these problems, you must decide which giving set would be the most appropriate.

Work out the drip rates for the following:

G.1 500 ml of sodium chloride 0.9% over 6 hours

G.2 500 ml of glucose 5% over 8 hours

G.3 100 ml of sodium chloride 0.9% over 1 hour

G.4 1 litre of glucose 4% and sodium chloride 0.18% over 12 hours

G.5 1 unit of blood (500 ml) over 4 hours

G.6 1 unit of blood (500 ml) over 6 hours

G.7 You need to give 3 litres of sodium chloride 0.9% over 24 hours. You only have one litre bags of sodium chloride 0.9%. At what rate should each bag run?

G.8 You need to give 1 g cefotaxime in 50 ml sodium chloride 0.9% over 40 minutes. What is the rate in drops/min?

G.9 You need to give an infusion of erythromycin 1 g in 200 ml sodium chloride 0.9% over 60 minutes. The concentration of erythromycin should not be greater then 5 mg/ml.

(i) What is the concentration of erythromycin?
(ii) What is the rate in drops/min?

CONVERSION OF INFUSION RATES (ml/hour or ml/min) TO drops/min

Sometimes it may be necessary to convert from ml/hour to drops/min.

WORKED EXAMPLE

1,000 ml of sodium chloride 0.9% has to be given at a rate of 125 ml/hour. What is the rate in drops/min?

You decide to use a standard giving set (20 drops/ml).

Step 1
Once again, you are converting a volume to the number of drops and hours to minutes (your final answer is in drops/min).

Step 2
Convert hours to minutes, i.e.

$$125 \text{ ml/hour} = 125 \text{ ml/60 min}$$

If the rate is already in ml/min, then obviously there is no need to convert from hours to minutes.

Step 3
Calculate the number of ml per minute by dividing the rate by 60, i.e.

$$125 \text{ ml/60 min becomes } \frac{125}{60} \text{ ml in 1 min}$$

Step 4
Convert ml/min to drops/min by multiplying by the drip rate of the giving set (in this case 20 drops/ml):

$$\frac{125}{60} \times 20 = 41.67 \text{ drops/min (42 drops/min, approx.)}$$

Answer: For 1,000 ml of sodium chloride 0.9% to be given at 125 ml/hour, the infusion rate should be 42 drops/min using a standard giving set.

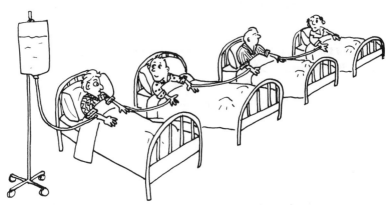

"I know they're supposed to cut costs, but this is ridiculous!"

A formula can be used:

$$\text{Drops/min} = \frac{\text{Hourly rate}}{60} \times \text{Drip rate for the giving set}$$

where in this case:

Hourly rate = 125 ml/hour
Drip rate for the giving set = 20 drops/ml
60 = number of minutes in an hour (converts hours to minutes)

Substitute the numbers in the formula:

$$\frac{125}{60} \times 20 = 41.67 \text{ drops/min} \ (42 \text{ drops/min, approx.})$$

Answer: For 1,000 ml of sodium chloride 0.9% to be given at 125 ml/hour, the infusion rate should be 42 drops/min using a standard giving set.

N.B. If the infusion rate is given as ml/min instead of ml/hour, then the formula will have to be rewritten:

$$\text{Drops/min} = \text{Rate (ml/min)} \times \text{Drip rate for the giving set}$$

You may have noticed that the volume of the infusion is not needed in the above calculation. This is because it is the *rate* of the infusion that is important which is the same irrespective of the volume. Therefore the volume can be ignored.

CONVERSION OF INFUSION RATES TO drops/min – SUMMARY

Conversion of ml/hour to drops/min

$$\text{Drops/min} = \frac{\text{Hourly rate}}{60} = \text{Drip rate for the giving set}$$

Conversion of ml/min to drops/min:

$$\text{Drops/min} = \text{Rate (ml/min)} \times \text{Drip rate for the giving set}$$

PROBLEMS

Work out the following drip rates:

G.10 Sodium chloride 0.9% at a rate of 4 ml/min
G.11 Glucose 5% at a rate of 120 ml/hour
G.12 Sodium chloride 0.9% at a rate of 3 ml/min
G.13 Glucose 5% at a rate of 167 ml/hour
G.14 One unit of blood (500 ml) at a rate of 125 ml/hour
G.15 Sodium chloride 0.9% at a rate of 250 ml/hour

CONVERSION OF DOSAGES TO INFUSION RATES (ml/hour AND drops/min)

Dosages can be expressed in many ways: mg/min or mcg/min and mg/kg/min or mcg/kg/min; and it may be necessary to convert to drops/min or ml/hour when using infusion pumps.

There are several types of infusion pumps available; the most commonly used pump is a volumetric pump (expressed in ml/hour). Therefore the only conversion you will probably need to do would be to ml/hour. However, there may be some drip rate pumps still in use, although the Department of Health does not recommend their use. Drip rate controllers (drops/min) and volumetric controllers (ml/hour) – pumps that rely on gravity – can still be used, though they are not considered very accurate. The following example shows the various steps in this type of calculation, and this can be adapted to any dosage for infusion rate calculation.

WORKED EXAMPLE

You have an infusion of dopamine 800 mg in 500 ml. The dose required is 2 mcg/kg/min for a patient weighing 68 kg.

 (i) What is the rate in ml/hour?
(ii) What is the rate in drops/min?

(i) Rate in ml/hour

Step 1
When carrying out this type of calculation, it is best to convert the dose required to a volume (in ml).

Step 2
First calculate the volume for 1 mcg of drug. It is best to work in micrograms since the dose is in micrograms: mcg/kg/min.

If the dose is in milligrams, then calculate the concentration of drug in mg/ml.

You have 800 mg in 500 ml; convert to micrograms, so this is equal to:

$$800 \text{ mg} \times 1{,}000 = 800{,}000 \text{ mcg in } 500 \text{ ml}$$

Thus the volume for 1 mcg is:

$$\frac{500}{800{,}000} \text{ ml}$$

Step 3
Now calculate the dose required:

Dose required = Patient's weight × Dose prescribed
$$= 68 \times 2 = 136 \text{ mcg/min}$$

If the dose is given as a total dose and not on a weight basis, then miss out this step.

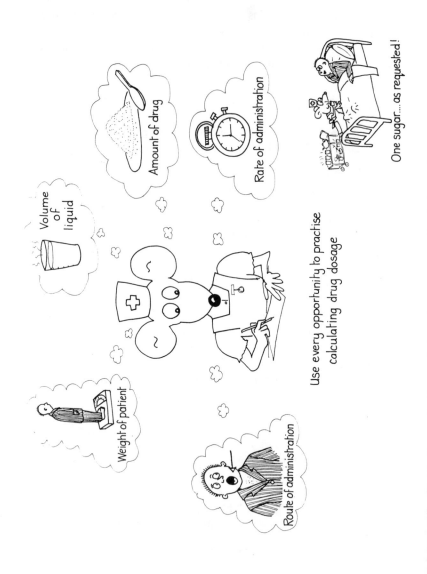

Step 4

The next step is to calculate the volume for the dose required. You have already worked out that the volume of 1 mcg of drug is:

$$\frac{500}{800,000} \, ml$$

Thus for the dose of 136 mcg, the volume is equal to:

$$\frac{500}{800,000} \times 136 \, ml = 0.085 \, ml$$

You can therefore rewrite the dose of 136 mcg/min as 0.085 ml/min. You have just converted the dose (136 mcg) to a volume (0.085 ml).

Step 5

You have just calculated that the rate to be given equals 0.085 ml/min. To calculate the rate in ml/hour, simply multiply by 60. This converts minutes to hours:

$$0.085 \, ml/min = 0.085 \times 60 = 5.1 \, ml/hour \, (5 \, ml/hour, \, approx.)$$

Answer: The rate required = 5 ml/hour.

If using a formula:

$$ml/hour = \frac{Total \; volume \; to \; be \; infused}{Total \; amount \; of \; drug} \times Dose$$

$$\times \, Weight \times 60$$

N.B. The dose and the total amount of drug must be in the *same units*, i.e. both in milligrams or micrograms.

In this case:

Total volume to be infused = 500 ml
Total amount of drug (mcg) = 800,000 mcg
Dose = 2 mcg/kg/min
Patient's weight = 68 kg
60 converts minutes to hours

Substitute the numbers in the formula:

$$\frac{500 \times 2 \times 68 \times 60}{800,000} = 5.1 \text{ ml/hour (5 ml/hour, approx.)}$$

Answer: The rate required = 5 ml/hour.

If the dose is given as a total dose and not on a weight basis, then the patient's weight is not needed:

$$\text{ml/hour} = \frac{\text{Total volume to be infused}}{\text{Total amount of drug}} \times \text{Dose} \times 60$$

(ii) Rate in drops/min

It is unlikely that the dosage of dopamine would ever need to be converted to drop/min (drip rate controllers are not considered very accurate), but this is included here for the purpose of practice.

Step 1
When carrying out this type of calculation, it is best to convert the dose required to a volume in ml, and then convert that volume to the 'number of drops' required.

Steps 2 to 4
Follow steps 2 to 4 as for ml/hour.

Step 5
Now calculate the rate (in drops/min) by multiplying the volume from step 4 by the drip rate of the giving set.
  You are using a microdrop giving set (60 drops/ml):

$$0.085 \text{ ml} \times 60 = 5.1 \text{ drops/min (5 drops/min, approx.)}$$

You have just converted the volume/min to drops/min.

Answer: The rate required is 5 drops/min using a microdrop giving set.

If using a formula:

$$\text{Drops/min} = \frac{\text{Total volume to be infused}}{\text{Total amount of drug}} \times \text{Dose}$$

$$\times \text{Weight} \times \text{Drip rate of set}$$

N.B. The dose and the total amount of drug must be in the *same units*, i.e. both in milligrams or micrograms.

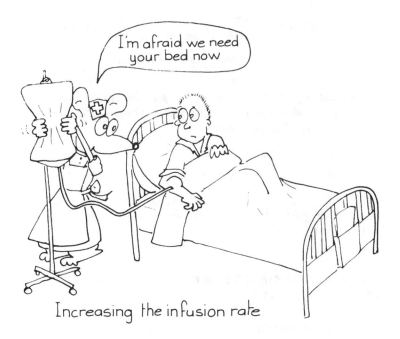

Increasing the infusion rate

In this case:

Total volume to be infused = 500 ml
Total amount of drug (mcg) = 800,000 mcg
Dose = 2 mcg/kg/min
Patient's weight = 68 kg
Drip rate of the giving set = 60 drops/ml

Substitute the numbers in the formula:

$$\frac{500 \times 2 \times 68 \times 60}{800,000} = 5.1 \text{ drops /min (5 drops/min, approx.)}$$

Answer: The rate required is 5 drops/min using a microdrop giving set.

If the dose is given as a total dose and not on a weight basis, then the patient's weight is not needed:

$$\text{Drops/min} = \frac{\text{Total volume to be infused}}{\text{Total amount of drug}} \times \text{Dose}$$

$$\times \text{ Drip rate of giving set}$$

As you can see from the above example, the answer for the rate in ml/hour and drops/min is the same. This is because you are multiplying by 60 in both cases:

60 converts minutes to hours (60 min = 1 hour)

60 drops/ml is the drip rate for a microdrop giving set

This is only true if you are using a microdrop giving set with a drip rate of 60 drops/ml. If using a different giving set, then the answers will *not* be the same.

CONVERSION OF DOSAGES TO INFUSION RATES – SUMMARY

Conversion of dose/kg weight to ml/hour:

$$\text{ml/hour} = \frac{\text{Total volume to be infused}}{\text{Total amount of drug}} \times \text{Dose} \times \text{Weight} \times 60$$

Conversion of total dose to ml/hour:

$$\text{ml/hour} = \frac{\text{Total volume to be infused}}{\text{Total amount of drug}} \times \text{Dose} \times 60$$

N.B. The dose and the total amount of drug must be in the *same units*, i.e. both in milligrams or micrograms.

Conversion of dose/kg weight to drops/min:

$$\text{Drops/min} = \frac{\text{Total volume to be infused}}{\text{Total amount of drug}} \times \text{Dose}$$

$$\times \text{ Weight} \times \text{Drip rate of giving set}$$

Conversion of total dose to drops/min:

$$\text{Drops/min} = \frac{\text{Total volume to be infused}}{\text{Total amount of drug}} \times \text{Dose}$$
$$\times \text{Drip rate of giving set}$$

PROBLEMS

G.16 You have a 500 ml infusion containing 50 mg nitroglycerin.
A dose of 10 mcg/min is required.
  (i) What is the rate in ml/hour?
  (ii) What is the rate in drops/min?

G.17 You are asked to give 500 ml of lignocaine 0.2% in glucose
at a rate of 2 mg/min.
  (i) What is the rate in ml/hour?
  (ii) What is the rate in drops/min?

G.18 Dopamine (200 mg in 50 ml) is being given by a syringe
driver. The dose required is 3 mcg/kg/min for a patient
weighing 80 kg. What is the rate in ml hour?

G.19 You have an isoprenaline infusion 5 mg in 500 ml glucose
5%. A dose of 5 mcg/min is required.
  (i) What is the rate in ml/hour?
  (ii) What is the rate in drops/min?

G.20 Nitroprusside is to be given to a 60 kg patient at a starting
rate of 2 mcg/kg/min. You have an infusion of 50 mg in
100 ml glucose 5%.
  (i) What is the rate in ml/hour?
  (ii) What is the rate in drops/min?

G.21 Glyceryl trinitrate is to be given at a starting rate of
150 mcg/min. You have an infusion of 50 mg in 500 ml
glucose 5%.
  (i) What is the rate in ml/hour?
  (ii) What is the rate in drops/min?

G.22 You have an infusion of frusemide 250 mg in 250 ml
sodium chloride 0.9%. The patient is to receive a dose of
1.5 mg/min.
  (i) What is the rate in ml/hour?

    (ii) What is the rate in drops/min?

G.23 You need to give an infusion of salbutamol. You have an ampoule containing salbutamol 5 mg in 5 ml which has to be added to a 500 ml infusion of sodium chloride 0.9%. The rate at which it has to be given is 5 mcg/min.

    (i) What is the concentration (mcg/ml) of salbutamol?

    (ii) What is the rate in ml/hour?

    (iii) what is the rate in drops/min?

G.24 You are asked to give an infusion of dobutamine to a patient weighing 73 kg at a dose of 5 mcg/kg/min. You have an infusion of 500 ml sodium chloride 0.9% containing one 250 mg vial of dobutamine.

    (i) What is the dose required (mcg/min)?

    (ii) What is the concentration (mcg/ml) of dobutamine?

    (iii) What is the rate in ml/hour?

    (iv) What is the rate in drops/min?

G.25 You are asked to give an infusion of isosorbide dinitrate 50 mg in 500 ml of glucose 5% at a rate of 2 mg/hour.

Adding a drug to the infusion

(i) What is the rate in ml/hour?
(ii) What is the rate in drops/min?
The rate is then changed to 5 mg/hour.
(iii) What is the new rate in ml/hour?
(iv) What is the new rate in drops/min?

CONVERSION OF ml/hour TO DOSAGES

It may be necessary to convert ml/hour back to the dose (mg/min or mcg/min; mg/kg/min or mcg/kg/min) for the purpose of checking that the infusion pump is giving the correct dose.

This will be done at varying frequencies depending upon local policies.

WORKED EXAMPLE

An infusion pump containing 250 mg dobutamine in 50 ml is running at a rate of 3.5 ml/hour. You want to convert to mcg/kg/min to check that the pump is set correctly. The patient's weight is 70 kg.

Step 1
In this type of calculation, convert the volume being given to the amount of drug, and then work out the amount of drug being given per minute or even per kilogram of the patient's weight.

Step 2
Convert the amount of drug (dobutamine) from milligrams to micrograms. The final answer wanted is in micrograms (mcg/kg/min), so convert everything to micrograms.

$$250 \text{ mg} = 250 \times 1,000 = 250,000 \text{ mcg}$$

Obviously, if the dose is already in milligrams, miss out this step.

Step 3
You have just worked out that you have 250,000 mcg of dobutamine in 50 ml. Now it is necessary to work out the amount in 1 ml:

250,000 mcg in 50 ml

$$\frac{250,000}{50} \text{ mcg in 1 ml}$$

Step 4
The rate at which the pump is running is 3.5 ml/hour. You have just worked out the amount in 1 ml (step 2), therefore for 3.5 ml:

$$3.5 \text{ ml/hour} = \frac{250,000}{50} \times 3.5 \text{ mcg/hour}$$

So the rate (ml/hour) has been converted to the amount of drug being given over an hour.

Step 5
In step 4, it was calculated that the rate is:

$$\frac{250,000}{50} \times 3.5 \text{ mcg/hour}$$

Now calculate the rate per minute by dividing by 60 (to convert hours to minutes):

$$\frac{250,000 \times 3.5}{50 \times 60} \text{ mcg/min}$$

Step 6
The final step in the calculation is to work out the rate according to the patient's weight (70 kg). If the dose is not given in terms of the patient's weight, then miss out this final step.

$$\frac{250,000 \times 3.5}{50 \times 60 \times 70} = 4.11 \text{ mcg/kg/min}$$

This can be 'rounded down' to 4 mcg/kg/min.

Now check your answer against the dose written on the drug chart to see if the pump is delivering the correct dose.

If your answer does not match the dose written on the drug chart, then re-check your calculation. If the answer is still the same, then inform the doctor and, if necessary, calculate the correct rate.

If using a formula:

$$\text{mg or mcg/kg/min} = \frac{\text{Rate (ml/hour)} \times \text{Amount of drug (mg or mcg)}}{60 \times \text{Weight (kg)} \times \text{Volume (ml)}}$$

N.B. If the dose is in milligrams, then the amount of drug must be in milligrams. If the dose is in micrograms, then the amount of drug must be in micrograms.

In this case:

Rate $= 3.5$ ml/hour
Amount of drug (mcg) $= 250,000$ mcg
Weight (kg) $= 70$ kg
Volume (ml) $= 50$ ml
60 converts hours to minutes

Substitute the numbers in the formula:

$$\frac{3.5 \times 250,000}{60 \times 70 \times 50} = 4.11 \text{ mcg/kg/min}$$

This can be 'rounded down' to 4 mcg/kg/min.

If the dose is in either mg/min or mcg/min, then the formula is now rewritten as:

$$\text{mg or mcg/min} = \frac{\text{Rate (ml/hour)} \times \text{Amount of drug (mg or mcg)}}{60 \times \text{Volume (ml)}}$$

N.B. If the dose is in milligrams, then the amount of drug must be in milligrams. If the dose is in micrograms, then the amount of drug must be in micrograms.

CONVERSION OF ml/hour TO DOSAGES – SUMMARY

Conversion of ml/hour to mg or mcg/kg/min:

$$\text{mg or mcg/kg/min} = \frac{\text{Rate (ml/hour)} \times \text{Amount of drug}}{60 \times \text{Weight (kg)} \times \text{Volume (ml)}}$$

Conversion of ml/hour to mg or mcg/min:

$$\text{mg or mcg/min} = \frac{\text{Rate (ml/hour)} \times \text{Amount of drug}}{60 \times \text{Volume (ml)}}$$

N.B. In both cases above, if the dose is in milligrams, then the amount of drug must be in milligrams; if the dose is in micrograms, then the amount of drug must be in micrograms.

PROBLEMS

Convert the following infusion pump rates to a mcg/kg/min dose:

G.26 You have dopamine 200 mg in 50 ml and the rate at which the pump is running = 4 ml/hour. The prescribed dose is 3 mcg/kg/min. The patient's weight is 89 kg. What dose is the pump delivering? If the dose is wrong, at which rate should the pump be set?

G.27 You have dobutamine 250 mg in 50 ml and the rate at which the pump is running = 5.6 ml/hour. The prescribed dose is 6 mcg/kg/min. The patient's weight is 64 kg. What dose is the pump delivering? If the dose is wrong, at which rate should the pump be set?

G.28 You have dopexamine 50 mg in 50 ml and the rate at which the pump is running = 2.3 ml/hour. The prescribed dose is 0.5 mcg/kg/min. The patient's weight is 78 kg. What dose is the pump delivering? If the dose is wrong, at which rate should the pump be set?

Convert the following infusion pump rates to a mg/min dose:

G.29 You have a 100 ml infusion containing 250 mg of frusemide being given by an infusion pump at a rate of 50 ml/hour.

The maximum rate at which frusemide can be given is 4 mg/min. At what rate is the pump delivering (mg/min)?

G.30 You have a 500 ml infusion of lignocaine 0.2% being given by an infusion pump at a rate of 90 ml/hour. The prescribed dose is 3 mg/min. What dose is the pump delivering (mg/min)?

G.31 You have a 500 ml infusion containing 2 mg of isoprenaline being given by an infusion pump at a rate of 45 ml/hour. The prescribed dose is 3 mcg/min. At what rate is the pump delivering (mcg/min)?

CALCULATING THE LENGTH OF TIME FOR I.V. INFUSIONS

Sometimes it may be necessary to calculate the number of hours an infusion should run at a specified rate. Also, this is a good way of checking your calculated drip rate for an infusion.

For example, you need to give a litre of 5% glucose over 8 hours. You have calculated that the drip rate should be 42 drops/min (using a standard giving set: 20 drops/ml).

To check your answer, you can calculate how long the infusion should take at the calculated drip rate of 42 drops/min. If your answers do not correspond (the answer should be 8 hours) then you have made an error and should re-check your calculation.

Alternatively, you can use this type of calculation to check the drip rate of an infusion already running.

EXAMPLE

If an infusion is supposed to run over 6 hours, and the infusion is nearly finished after 4 hours, you can check the drip rate by calculating how long the infusion should take using that drip rate. If the calculated answer is less than 6 hours, then the original drip rate was wrong and the doctor should be informed, if necessary. This is particularly important if a drug has been added to the infusion – some drugs have an adverse effect if infused too fast.

WORKED EXAMPLE

The doctor prescribes 1 litre of 5% glucose to be given over 8 hours. The drip rate for the infusion is calculated to be 40 drops/min. You wish to check the drip rate. How many hours is the infusion going to run?

(Standard giving set = 20 drops/ml.)

Step 1

In this calculation, you first convert the volume being infused to drops, then calculate how long it will take at the specified rate.

Step 2

First, convert the volume to drops by multiplying the volume of the infusion by the number of drops/ml for the giving set:

$1{,}000 \times 20 = 20{,}000$ drops

Step 3

From the rate, calculate how many minutes it will take for 1 drop, i.e.

40 drops per minute

$$1 \text{ drop} = \frac{1}{40} \text{ min}$$

Step 4

Calculate how many minutes it will take to infuse the total number of drops:

$$1 \text{ drop} = \frac{1}{40} \text{ min}$$

$$20{,}000 \text{ drops} = \frac{1}{40} \times 20{,}000 = 500 \text{ min}$$

Step 5

Convert minutes to hours by dividing by 60:

$$500 \text{ min} = \frac{500}{60} = 8.333 \text{ hours}$$

How much is 0.333 of an hour? Multiply by 60 to convert part of an hour back to minutes:

$$0.333 \times 60 = 20 \text{ min}$$

Answer: 1 litre of glucose 5% at a rate of 40 drops/min will take 8 hours 20 min to run.

A formula can be used:

$$\text{Number of hours the infusion is to run} = \frac{\text{Volume of the infusion}}{\text{Rate (drops/min)} \times 60} \times \text{Drip rate of giving set}$$

where in this case:

Volume of the infusion = 1,000 ml
Rate (drops/min) = 40 drops/min
Drip rate of giving set = 20 drops/ml
60 converts minutes to hours

Substitute the numbers in the formula:

$$\frac{1,000}{40 \times 60} \times 20 = 8.333 \text{ hours}$$

Convert 0.333 hours to minutes = 20 min.

Answer: 1 litre of glucose 5% at a rate of 40 drops/min will take 8 hours 20 min to run.

N.B. If the infusion is being given over a number of minutes, then the formula can be rewritten as:

$$\text{Number of minutes the infusion is to run} = \frac{\text{Volume of the infusion}}{\text{Rate (drops/min)}} \times \text{Drip rate of giving set}$$

CALCULATING THE LENGTH OF TIME FOR I.V. INFUSIONS – SUMMARY

Infusion being given over a number of hours:

$$\text{Number of hours the infusion is to run} = \frac{\text{Volume of the infusion}}{\text{Rate (drops/min)} \times 60} \times \text{Drip rate of giving set}$$

Infusion being given over a number of minutes:

$$\text{Number of minutes the infusion is to run} = \frac{\text{Volume of the infusion}}{\text{Rate (drops/min)}} \times \text{Drip rate of giving set}$$

PROBLEMS

G.32 A 1 litre infusion of sodium chloride 0.9% is being given over 16 hours using a standard giving set. The rate at which the infusion is being run is 21 drops/min. How long will the infusion run at the specified rate?

G.33 A 100 ml infusion of sodium chloride 0.9% is being given over 60 minutes using a standard giving set. The rate at which the infusion is being run is 30 drops/min. How long will the infusion run at the specified rate?

G.34 A unit of blood (500 ml) is being given over 4 hours using a standard giving set. The rate at which the infusion is being run is 30 drops/min. How long will the infusion run at the specified rate?

G.35 (i) A 500 ml infusion of sodium chloride 0.9% is being given over 8 hours using a standard giving set. The rate at which the infusion is being run is 20 drops/min. How long will the infusion run at the specified rate?

(ii) After 4 hours, the rate is changed to 30 drops/min. How long will the remaining infusion run at the new rate?

G.36 You have a 100 ml infusion containing 250 mg of frusemide running at a rate of 42 drops/min. The maximum rate allowed for frusemide is 4 mg/min.

(i) How long should the infusion take if the maximum rate of 4 mg/min is not to be exceeded?

(ii) Is the rate at which the infusion is currently being given correct?

G.37 You have a 200 ml infusion containing 1 g of vancomycin running at a rate of 50 drops/min. The maximum rate allowed for vancomycin is 10 mg/min, otherwise the patient will experience an allergic type reaction (known as 'red man' syndrome).

   (i) How long should the infusion take if the maximum rate of 10 mg/min is not to be exceeded?

   (ii) Is the rate at which the infusion is currently being given correct?

I.V. INFUSION THERAPY

I.V. infusions are a common sight on hospital wards, and the majority of patients will have I.V. infusions as a part of their treatment.

Intravenous fluids should not be considered simply as a means of administering drugs or as plasma expanders. Inappropriate use can lead to imbalances in electrolytes, acid–base disturbances, and fluid imbalances.

However, water has an important role in the normal function of the body. Its major function is as a transport system for nutrients and waste products. Also the kidneys require a minimum of 500 ml to maintain normal renal function, and the lung surface must be 'wet' to allow gaseous exchange. Water is also important in the maintenance of blood volume. Therefore, it is essential to ensure an adequate fluid balance.

Fluid balance in the body

There is a balance between intake and loss:

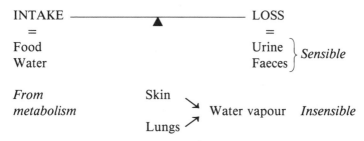

TABLE 9.1 Average adult water loss per day

	Range (ml/day)	Average (ml/day)	Daily losses (%)
Insensible losses			
Skin	400–700	550	21%
Lungs	300–600	400	15%
Sensible losses			
Faeces	100–200	150	6%
Urine	500–3,000	1,500	58%
		2,600	100%

It is difficult to predict the daily water loss for an average person since there can be a large range in the water loss per day. However, average adult water loss per day is shown in Table 9.1.

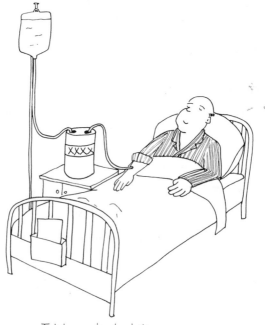

Total parenteral nutrition

It is accepted that the average loss is around 2,500–2,600 ml per day. Obviously, this can only be used as a guide, several factors can alter daily losses. For example, pyrexia can increase water loss from the skin and lungs dramatically.

There are various methods for calculating daily fluid requirements.

One method assumes that approximately 30 ml/kg/day is required for maintenance of fluid balance. This method does not take into account the variation of fluid requirements with age (children require more fluid per kilogram body weight than adults).

A second method uses body surface area and this is more accurate with regard to age. Approximately 1,500 ml/m^2/day is required for maintenance of daily fluid requirements.

If you are using body weight, then from Table 9.1 roughly two-thirds are sensible losses (urine and faeces, 64%) and one-third is insensible losses (skin and lungs, 36%). If using 30 ml/kg/day as a means of calculation, then sensible losses are approximately 20 ml/kg/day and insensible losses are approximately 10 ml/kg/day.

Therefore it is possible to calculate fluid loss on a weight basis. With obese patients, it is best to estimate fluid loss on Ideal Body Weight (I.B.W).

Fluid loss estimation

(a) Insensible fluid loss (from skin and lungs) is estimated as 10 ml/kg/day:

Daily loss = 10 ml/kg/day (10 × body weight)

(b) Sensible fluid loss (in urine and faeces) is estimated as 20 ml/kg/day:

Daily loss = 20 ml/kg/day (20 × body weight)

Urine loss can vary greatly: it depends upon fluid intake and renal function. It is best to have a 24 hour urine collection, but if this is not possible, then it can be estimated on a body weight basis.

However, if urine loss is being measured, the loss in the faeces will have to be taken into account separately. Approximately, at least 50% of the stool must be water to avoid constipation. So average water loss is 150 ml/day.

Total estimated fluid loss

Estimated daily loss = Insensible losses + Sensible losses
= $(10 \, \text{ml/kg/day})$ + $(20 \, \text{ml/kg/day})$

This total daily water loss is the amount that should be given every day to prevent dehydration.

However, correction of existing imbalances should be addressed. This means measuring and replacing unusual fluid losses, such as those caused by diuresis, vomiting, burns, fever, diarrhoea, G.I. disturbances, drains or 'third-spacing' (i.e. shifts in fluids as in ascites). This is achieved by doing daily weights (1 kg is approximately 1 litre) and accurate measurement of fluid intake and output.

Total volume to = Estimation of + Volume of losses during
be given daily   daily loss   the preceding 24 hours

Electrolyte requirements

The daily electrolyte requirements can be estimated and then adjusted according to plasma levels.

Sodium

The normal intake is approximately 150 mmol/day and, assuming that an average man weighs 70 kg, the approximate requirement is 2 mmol/kg/day:

Daily sodium requirement = 2 mmol/kg/day (2 × body weight)

Potassium

The normal intake is approximately 65 mmol/day and, assuming that an average man weighs 70 kg, the approximate requirement is 1 mmol/kg/day:

Daily potassium requirement = 1 mmol/kg/day (1 × body weight)

Simple infusion fluid regimens

When deciding on an I.V. fluid regimen, calculate the daily fluid and electrolyte requirements and then adjust to the patient's individual requirements.

Once calculated, the most appropriate fluid must be chosen to meet the patient's needs.

It is not necessary to have an infusion regimen that meets the patient's requirements exactly. It is normal to have a regimen that provides approximate amounts to the calculated daily fluid, sodium and potassium requirements using standard infusion bags.

Some doctors have their own infusion regimens for certain patients which will not follow this regimen exactly.

EXAMPLE 1: A 90 kg patient

Fluid requirements
Insensible losses = (10 × body weight) ml = 10 × 90 =   900 ml
Sensible losses   = (20 × body weight) ml = 20 × 90 = 1,800 ml

                                                       2,700 ml

Electrolyte requirements
Sodium   = (2 × body weight) mmol = 2 × 90 = 180 mmol.
Potassium   = (1 × body weight) mmol = 1 × 90 =   90 mmol.

Infusion fluid regimen
Fluid required   = approx. 2.5 litres (2,500 ml).
Sodium required   = approx. 150 mmol (content of 1 litre
                        sodium chloride 0.9%).
Potassium required = approx. 80 mmol (max. in 1 litre =
40 mmol, therefore give in 2 litres).

Therefore you need to give 2.5 litres, 1 litre being sodium chloride 0.9%, with 40 mmol of potassium per litre:

Potassium 0.3% + sodium chloride 0.9%, 1 litre (150 mmol sodium, 40 mmol potassium)
Potassium 0.3% + glucose 5%, 1 litre (40 mmol potassium)
Glucose 5%, 500 ml

EXAMPLE 2: A 78 kg patient (urine output = 1,000 ml)

Fluid requirements
Insensible losses = (10 × body weight) ml = 10 × 78 =   780 ml
Urine losses = 1,000 ml (measured)   1,000 ml
Faeces = 150 ml   150 ml

                                                       1,930 ml

Electrolyte requirements
Sodium = (2 × body weight) mmol = 2 × 78 = 156 mmol.
Potassium = (1 × body weight) mmol = 1 × 78 = 78 mmol.

Infusion fluid regimen
Fluid required = approx. 2 litres (2,000 ml).
Sodium required = approx. 150 mmol (content of 1 litre
                 sodium chloride 0.9%).
Potassium required = approx. 80 mmol (max. in 1 litre =
40 mmol, therefore give in 2 litres).

Therefore you need to give 2 litres, each containing 40 mmol
of potassium, of which 1 litre is sodium chloride 0.9%:

Potassium 0.3% + sodium chloride 0.9%, 1 litre
(150 mmol sodium, 40 mmol potassium)

Potassium 0.3% + glucose 5%, 1 litre
(40 mmol potassium)

These are only estimates – fluid regimens will be prescribed to
individual patient requirements.

PAEDIATRIC INFUSION REGIMENS

Fluid and electrolyte balance in a child can be complex, but the same
factors seen in adults apply to children.

   Fluid requirements appear relatively higher than in adults because
rate of fluid metabolism corresponds to surface area rather than
body weight. In fact, fluid requirements in children and adults are
identical when expressed per surface area.

   Fluid losses in children are difficult to predict, but gains and
losses can be estimated on a body surface area basis. Average water
loss per day in children is shown in Table 9.2.

Estimation of fluid requirements

There are several ways of estimating normal requirements: surface
area correlates the best, but body weight is the easiest method to use.

TABLE 9.2 Average child water loss per day

	Average $(ml/m^2/day)$	Daily losses (%)
Insensible losses		
Skin	775	21%
Lungs		15%
Sensible losses		
Faeces	100	6%
Urine	875	58%
	1,750	100%
Sources		
From metabolism	250	
Total requirement	1,500	

(a) Body surface area

Only really works for children weighing more than 10 kg:

Normal daily requirements = $1,500 \, ml/m^2/day$

(b) Body weight

Depending upon which reference book you use, the figures can vary slightly. However, the general rule is:

100 ml/kg for the *first* 10 kg
50 ml/kg for the *next* 10 kg
20 ml/kg for every kilogram above 20 kg

For example, for a 25 kg child:

100 ml/kg × 10 kg = 1,000 ml for the first 10 kg
50 ml/kg × 10 kg = 500 ml for the next 10 kg
20 ml/kg × 5 kg = 100 ml for every kg above 20 kg

25 kg 1,600 ml

For neonates (full term), the average fluid requirements are:

Day 1	60 ml/kg/day
Day 2	90 ml/kg/day
Day 3	120 ml/kg/day
Day 4+	150 ml/kg/day

For premature neonates, the fluid requirements vary. See a neonatal reference book for guidance.

Estimation of electrolyte requirements

The daily electrolyte requirements can be estimated and then adjusted according to the patient's requirements.

Sodium

The requirements for a child can vary, but the general figure is:

3 mmol/kg/day

TABLE 9.3 Electrolyte content of common infusions

	Sodium (mmol/L)	Potassium* (mmol/L)	Energy (kcal/L)
Sodium chloride 0.9%	150	0	0
Glucose 5%	0	0	200
Sodium chloride 0.18% + Glucose 4%	30	0	160
Sodium chloride 0.9% + Potassium 0.3%	150	40	0
Sodium chloride 0.9% + Potassium 0.15%	150	20	0
Potassium 0.3% + Glucose 5%	0	40	200
Potassium 0.15% + Glucose 5%	0	20	200
Potassium 0.15% + Sodium chloride 0.18% + Glucose 4%	30	20	160
Potassium 0.3% + Sodium chloride 0.18% + Glucose 4%	30	40	160

* Maximum amount of potassium in 1 litre = 40 mmol.

Potassium
The requirements for a child can vary, but the general figure is:

2 mmol/kg/day

As before, the above estimations can only be considered as a guide.
Requirements are usually adjusted to individual needs.

Syringe drivers and pumps

OBJECTIVES
At the end of this section you should be familiar with the following:
Syringe drivers
  Calculation of dose

How to set the rate
How to increase the dose
Syringe pumps
Heparin
Insulin
Other drugs

SYRINGE DRIVERS

These pumps are designed to deliver drugs accurately over a certain
period of time (usually 24 hours). They have the advantage of being
small and compact, can be carried easily by the patient, and avoid
the need for numerous injections throughout the day. These pumps
are useful for potent drugs or small doses of drugs that have to
be administered accurately, for example opiates, insulin, chemo-
therapy, hormones and anti-emetics.
  There are two types of syringe drivers:

1. Those designed to deliver drugs at a daily rate (i.e. over 24
   hours)
2. Those designed to deliver drugs at an hourly rate.

There are a number of syringe drivers available. The Graseby MS
Series are the most widely used, and these are given as an example
here. When using other types, you should check the User's Manual
for rate calculations. Figure 9.1 shows the Graseby MS16A syringe
driver.

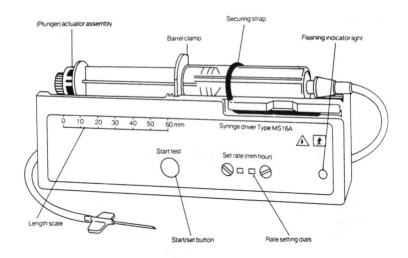

FIGURE 9.1 The Graseby Medical MS16A syringe driver. (From: *The Royal Marsden Hospital Manual of Clinical Nursing Procedures*, 2nd edn, 1990, London, Harper & Row)

Calculation of dose

The amount required is the total dose to be given over 24 hours.

(a) If the dose is prescribed as 'mg/hour', then it is necessary to calculate the total amount for 24 hours by multiplying by 24, i.e. if the dose is 3 mg/hour, then:

Total amount required for 24 hours = $3 \times 24 = 72$ mg

(b) If the dose is prescribed every 4 hours (or whatever), multiply the dose by the number of times the dose is given in 24 hours. For example, 20 mg every 4 hours. The dose is being given 6 times in 24 hours (divide 24 by the dosing frequency, i.e. $\frac{24}{4} = 6$):

Total amount required for 24 hours = $20 \times 6 = 120$ mg

(c) If the dose is prescribed as 'mg/day' (24 hours), then no calculation is necessary, i.e. if the dose is 60 mg/day (24 hours), then:

Total amount required for 24 hours = 60 mg

To set the rate

First, determine the 'fluid length' (*L*) of the volume in the syringe by measuring against the millimetre scale on the syringe driver (see Figure 9.2).

A 10 ml syringe will have an approximate 'fluid length' (*L*) of 48 mm.

Syringe drivers (mm/24 hours)

For a driver delivering at a daily rate (over 24 hours), set the dial to 48. So the dial should read: 48 mm/24 hours.

There is no calculation involved since the driver delivers the 'fluid length' (*L*) over 24 hours:

Dial setting (mm/24 hours) = 'Fluid length' (mm)

Syringe drivers (mm/hour)

For a driver delivering at an hourly rate, set the dial to 02. So the dial should read: 02 mm/hour.

Divide the 'fluid length' (*L*) by 24 to give the hourly rate:

$$\text{Dial setting (mm/hour)} = \frac{\text{'Fluid length' (mm)}}{24}$$

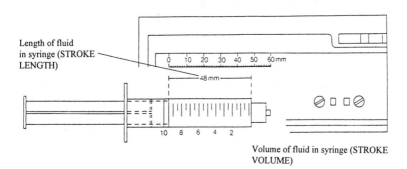

Length of fluid in syringe (STROKE LENGTH)

Volume of fluid in syringe (STROKE VOLUME)

FIGURE 9.2 Measurement of fluid length in syringe against millimetre scale on the syringe driver. (From: *The Royal Marsden Hospital Manual of Clinical Nursing Procedures*, 2nd edn, 1990, London, Harper & Row)

Increases in dose

Sometimes, when a patient is half-way through an infusion, it may be necessary to increase the dose. There are two ways of achieving this:

1. Stop the infusion and replace with a new syringe containing a higher dose.
2. Increase the rate.

Increasing the rate: drivers calibrated in mm/hour

Since this type of syringe driver is calibrated with an hourly rate, a small change in the rate will mean a very large increase in the dose over 24 hours; the rate, on the dial, is usually increased by increments of one.

When increasing the rate, you will have to calculate the new dose the patient is receiving. A formula can be used to do this:

$$\text{New dose} = \frac{\text{Original dose} \times \text{New rate}}{2}$$

EXAMPLE

You have a syringe containing 30 mg diamorphine and the current rate is 2 mm/hour (02 on the scale).

You increase the rate to 3 mm/hour (03 on the scale). The new dose the patient is receiving equals:

$$\text{New dose} = \frac{30 \times 3}{2} = 45 \text{ mg}$$

Therefore the patient is now receiving 45 mg over 24 hours.

You can only increase the dose by increasing the rate on the dial; it is very difficult to increase the actual dose and try to work out the new rate on the dial (i.e. increase the dose from 30 mg to 50 mg.

N.B. When you increase the rate, the syringe is being infused at a faster rate and consequently will not last for 24 hours.

Increasing the rate: drivers calibrated in mm/24 hours

Since this type of syringe driver is calibrated in terms of 24 hours, a small change in the rate will mean a very small increase in the dose over 24 hours; the rate, on the dial, is usually increased by increments of 12 or even 24.

Once again, when increasing the rate, you will have to calculate the new dose the patient is receiving. A formula can be used to do this:

$$\text{New dose} = \frac{\text{Original dose} \times \text{New rate}}{\text{Old rate}}$$

EXAMPLE

A patient is receiving 30 mg diamorphine over 24 hours and the current rate is 48 mm/24 hours (48 on the scale).

You increase the rate to 72 mm/24 hours (72 on the scale). This is an increase of 24. The new dose the patient is receiving equals:

$$\text{New dose} = \frac{30 \times 72}{48} = 45 \text{ mg}$$

Therefore the patient is now receiving 45 mg over 24 hours.

Note again that you can only increase the dose by increasing the rate on the dial; it is very difficult to increase the actual dose and try to work out the new rate on the dial (i.e. increase the dose from 30 mg to 50 mg).

N.B. When you increase the rate, the syringe is being infused at a faster rate and consequently will not last for 24 hours.

SYRINGE PUMPS

The commonest type of syringe pump used is a 50 ml syringe size. These are used for small volume infusions where smooth output and precise control are of prime importance. They are fairly simple to use and can be extremely accurate. Potent drugs (that need to be given accurately) are usually given this way.

Once again, to set up the system please read the Manufacturer's guidelines, but basically the principles are alike. See Figure 9.3.

This type of pump can be used for many drugs, but is most commonly used on the wards for heparin and insulin.

Heparin

Intravenous heparin is usually given via this type of pump, over 24 hours. Heparin is available in many different concentrations (e.g. 1,000 units and 5,000 units), which are diluted further with sodium chloride 0.9%.

To calculate the required amount, simply take ampoules containing the appropriate strengths of heparin and dilute to 48 ml. Then, simply give at a rate of 2 ml/hour, which ensures the dose is given over 24 hours.

EXAMPLE

24,000 units of heparin to be given over 24 hours.

Select

$$4 \times 5,000 \text{ units/ml} = 20,000 \text{ units in 4 ml}$$
$$4 \times 1,000 \text{ units/ml} = \underline{4,000 \text{ units in 4 ml}}$$
$$24,000 \text{ units in 8 ml}$$

Then add sodium chloride 0.9% to 48 ml. Therefore, draw up

$$4 \times 5,000 \text{ units (4 ml)}$$
$$+ \ 4 \times 1,000 \text{ units (4 ml)}$$
$$+ \ 40 \text{ ml sodium chloride 0.9\%}$$

in a 50 ml syringe and mix. Set the pump to 2 ml/hour, to give the 48 ml over 24 hours.

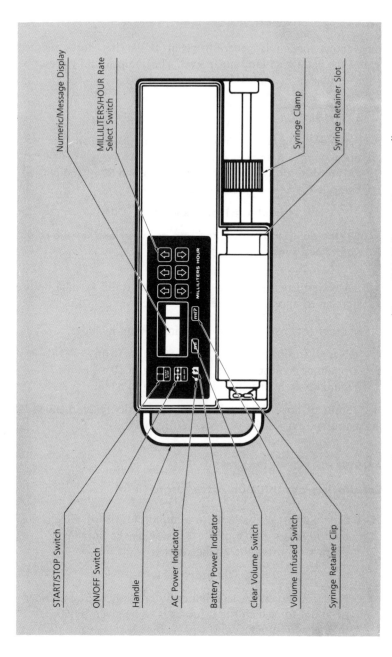

START/STOP Switch

ON/OFF Switch

Handle

AC Power Indicator

Battery Power Indicator

Clear Volume Switch

Volume Infused Switch

Syringe Retainer Clip

Numeric/Message Display

MILLILITERS/HOUR Rate
Select Switch

Syringe Clamp

Syringe Retainer Slot

FIGURE 9.3 Setting up a syringe pump. (From: IVAC* Corporation manual)

Insulin

Intravenous insulin is generally given at varying doses titrated against the patient's blood sugar level. The pumps usually prescribe 1 unit of insulin in 1 ml sodium chloride 0.9%.

EXAMPLE

A patient is to receive insulin at varying doses from 0.5 units/hour to 5 units/hour.

Therefore draw up 50 units of insulin and 50 ml sodium chloride 0.9% in a 50 ml syringe, to give:

1 unit of insulin = 1 ml of solution

Set the pump to the required rate as prescribed for the relevant blood sugar.

N.B. Always draw up insulin in a specific insulin syringe before transferring to another syringe for I.V. use.

Other drugs that can be given by syringe pump include:

Glyceryl trinitrate	50 mg in 50 ml
Dopamine hydrochloride	200 mg in 50 ml
Dobutamine hydrochloride	250 mg in 50 ml

N.B. Some of these dilutions are not necessarily recommended by the manufacturer – always check before giving.

ANSWERS TO PROBLEMS

Calculating I.V. infusion rates (drops/min)

G.1 First convert the volume to a number of drops. To do this, multiply the volume of the infusion by the number of drops per ml for the giving set, i.e.

$$500 \times 20 = 10,000 \text{ drops}$$

Next convert hours to minutes by multiplying the number of hours for which the infusion is to be given by 60 (60 minutes = 1 hour):

6 hours = 6 × 60 = 360 minutes

Write down what you have just calculated, i.e. the total number of drops to be given over how many minutes:

10,000 drops over 360 min

Calculate the number of drops per minute by dividing the number of drops by the number of minutes, i.e.

10,000 drops over 360 minutes

$$\frac{10,000}{360} = 27.78 \text{ drops/min (28 drops/min, approx.)}$$

Answer: To give 500 ml of sodium chloride 0.9% over 6 hours, the rate will have to be 28 drops/min using a standard giving set (20 drops/ml).

If using the formula:

$$\text{Drops/min} = \frac{\text{Drops/ml of the giving set} \times \text{Volume of the infusion}}{\text{Number of hours the infusion is to run} \times 60}$$

where in this case:

Drops/ml of the giving set (SGS) = 20 drops/ml
Volume of the infusion (in ml) = 500 ml
Number of hours the infusion is to run = 6 hours

substitute the numbers in the formula:

$$\frac{20 \times 500}{6 \times 60} = 27.78 \text{ drops/min (28 drops/min, approx.)}$$

Answer: To give 500 ml of sodium chloride 0.9% over 6 hours, the rate will have to be 28 drops/min using a standard giving set (20 drops/ml).

G.2 20.8 drops/min (21 drops/min) – SGS (20 drops/ml)
G.3 33.3 drops/min (33 drops/min) – SGS (20 drops/ml)
G.4 27.7 drops/min (28 drops/min) – SGS (20 drops/ml)
G.5 31.25 drops/min (31 drops/min) – SGS (15 drops/ml)
G.6 20.8 drops/min (21 drops/min) – SGS (20 drops/ml)
G.7 3 litres over 24 hours, thus 1 litre over $\frac{24}{3} = 8$ hours.

Answer: 41.67 drops/min (42 drops/min) – SGS (20 drops/ml)

G.8 Calculate the total number of drops required by multiplying:

Total volume × drip rate for the giving set
50 × 20 = 1,000 drops

Thus you are giving 1,000 drops over 40 minutes. Therefore:

$$\frac{1,000}{40} = 25 \text{ drops/min}$$

Answer: 25 drops/min – SGS (20 drops/ml)

If using the formula:

$$\text{Drops/min} = \frac{\text{Drops/ml of the giving set} \times \text{Volume of the infusion}}{\text{Number of minutes the infusion is to run}}$$

where in this case:

Drops/ml of the giving set (SGS) = 20 drops/ml
Volume of the infusion (in ml) = 50 ml
Number of minutes the infusion is to run = 40 min

substitute the numbers in the formula:

$$\frac{20 \times 50}{40} = 25 \text{ drops/min}$$

Answer: 25 drops/min – SGS (20 drops/ml)

G.9 (i) You have a 200 ml infusion of erythromycin 1 g (1,000 ml). To find the concentration (mg/ml), divide the amount of erythromycin by the volume, i.e.

$$\frac{1,000}{200} = 5 \text{ mg/ml}$$

Answer: The concentration of erythromycin equals 5 mg/ml.

(ii) Convert the volume to be infused to the number of drops by multiplying:

Total volume × drip rate for the giving set
200 × 20 = 4,000 drops

Thus it is 4,000 drops to be given over 60 minutes.

$$\frac{4,000}{60} = 66.67 \text{ drops/min (67 drops/min)}$$

Answer: The required rate = 67 drops/min using a standard giving set (20 drops/ml).

If using the formula:

$$\text{Drops/min} = \frac{\text{Drops/ml of the giving set × Volume of the infusion}}{\text{Number of minutes the infusion is to run}}$$

where in this case:

Drops/ml of the giving set (SGS)   = 20 drops/ml
Volume of the infusion (in ml)   = 200 ml
Number of minutes the infusion
is to run   = 60 min

substitute the numbers in the formula:

$$\frac{20 \times 200}{60} = 66.67 \text{ drops/min (67 drops/min)}$$

Answer: The required rate = 67 drops/min using a standard giving set (20 drops/ml).

Conversion of infusion rates to drops/min

G.10 The rate is already in ml/min, so there is no need to convert to ml/min. Convert ml/min to drops/min by multiplying by the drip rate of the giving set (in this case 20 drops/ml):

4 × 20 = 80 drops/min

Answer: The drip rate required = 80 drops/min using a standard giving set (20 drops/ml).

A formula can be used:

Drops/min = Rate (ml/min) × Drip rate for the giving set

where:

Rate (ml/min)   = 4 ml/min
Drip rate for the giving set = 20 drops/ml

Substitute the numbers in the formula:

4 × 20 = 80 drops/min

Answer: The drip rate required = 80 drops/min using a standard giving set (20 drops/ml).

G.11 Convert the rate from ml/hour to ml/min, i.e.

120 ml/hour equals 120 ml/60 min

Calculate the number of ml per minute by dividing by 60:

120 ml/60 min becomes $\frac{120}{60}$ ml/min

Convert ml/min to drops/min by multiplying by the drip rate of the giving set (in this case 20 drops/ml – SGS):

$\frac{120}{60} \times 20 = 40$ drops/min

Answer: 40 drops/min – SGS (20 drops/ml)

A formula can be used:

Drops/min = $\frac{\text{Hourly rate (ml/hour)}}{60} \times$ Drip rate for the giving set

where:

Hourly rate (ml/min)   = 120 ml/hour
Drip rate for the giving set = 20 drops/ml

Substitute the numbers in the formula:

$$\frac{120}{60} \times 20 = 40 \text{ drops/min}$$

Answer: 40 drops/min – SGS (20 drops/ml)

G.12 60 drops/min – SGS (20 drops/ml)

G.13 55.6 drops/min (56 drops/min). This can be 'rounded up' to make administration easier: 60 drops/min – SGS (20 drops/ml).

G.14 31.2 drops/min (31 drops/min). This can be 'rounded down' to make administration easier: 30 drops/min – SGS (20 drops/ml).

G.15 83.3 drops/min (83 drops/min). This can be 'rounded down' to make administration easier: 80 drops/min – SGS (20 drops/ml).

Conversion of dosages to infusion rates (ml/hour and drops/min)

G.16 (i) Rate in ml/hour

First convert the amount of drug from milligrams to micrograms (the dose is in micrograms, so it is best to work in micrograms):

Nitroglycerin 50 mg = 50 × 1,000 = 50,000 mcg

Next, calculate the volume for 1 mcg of nitroglycerin:

$$50,000 \text{ mcg in 500 ml; } 1 \text{ mcg} = \frac{500}{50,000} \text{ ml}$$

Thus for the dose of 10 mcg/min, this is equal to:

$$\frac{500}{50,000} \times 10 = 0.1 \text{ ml/min}$$

You have just calculated that the rate to be given = 0.1 ml/min. To calculate the rate in ml/hour, simply multiply by 60. This converts minutes to hours:

0.1 ml/min = 0.1 × 60 = 6 ml/hour

Answer: The rate required = 6 ml/hour.

If using the formula:

$$\text{ml/hour} = \frac{\text{Total volume to be infused}}{\text{Total amount of drug}} \times \text{Dose} \times 60$$

where:

Total volume to be infused   = 500 ml
Total amount of drug (mcg) = 50,000 mcg
Dose   = 10 mcg/min

substitute the numbers in the formula:

$$\frac{500 \times 10 \times 60}{50,000} = 6 \text{ ml/hour}$$

Answer: The rate required = 6 ml/hour.

(ii) Rate in drops/min

You have just calculated that the rate to be given = 0.1 ml/min. Now calculate the rate (in drops/min) by multiplying by the drip rate for the giving set. If using a microdrop giving set (60 drops/ml), then:

$$0.1 \text{ ml/min} = 0.1 \times 60 = 6 \text{ drops/min}$$

Answer: The rate required is 6 drops/min using a microdrop giving set (60 drops/ml).

If using the formula:

$$\text{Drops/min} = \frac{\text{Total volume to be infused}}{\text{Total amount of drug}} \times \text{Dose} \times \text{Drip rate of of the giving set}$$

where:

Total volume to be infused   = 500 ml
Total amount of drug (mcg) = 50,000 mcg
Dose   = 10 mcg/min
Drip rate of the giving set   = 60 drops/ml

substitute the numbers in the formula:

$$\frac{500 \times 10 \times 60}{50,000} = 6 \text{ drops/min}$$

Answer: The rate required is 6 drops/min using a microdrop giving set (60 drops/ml).

G.17 (i) 60 ml/hour

(ii) 20 drops/min – SGS (20 drops/ml)

60 drops/min – microdrop giving set (60 drops/ml)

G.18 First calculate the dose required:

$$\text{Dose required} = \text{Dose (3 mcg/kg/min)} \times \text{Patient's weight (80 kg)}$$
$$= 3 \times 80 = 240 \text{ mcg/min}$$

Convert the amount of drug from milligrams to micrograms (the dose is in micrograms, so it is best to work in micrograms):

Dopamine 200 mg $= 200 \times 1{,}000 = 200{,}000$ mcg

Next, calculate the volume for 1 mcg of dopamine:

$$200{,}000 \text{ mcg in 50 ml; } 1 \text{ mcg} = \frac{50}{200{,}000} \text{ ml}$$

Thus for the dose of 240 mcg/min, this is equal to:

$$\frac{50}{200{,}000} \times 240 = 0.06 \text{ ml/min}$$

You have just calculated that the rate to be given $=$ 0.06 ml/min. To calculate the rate in ml/hour, simply multiply by 60. This converts minutes to hours:

$$0.06 \text{ ml/min} = 0.06 \times 60 = 3.6 \text{ ml/hour}$$

Answer: The rate required $= 3.6$ ml/hour.

If using the formula:

$$\text{ml/hour} = \frac{\text{Total volume to be infused}}{\text{Total amount of drug}} \times \text{Dose} \times \text{Weight} \times 60$$

where:

Total volume to be infused $= 50$ ml

Total amount of drug (mcg) $= 200{,}000$ mcg

Dose $= 3$ mcg/kg/min

Patient's weight $= 80$ kg

substitute the numbers in the formula:

$$\frac{50 \times 3 \times 80 \times 60}{200,000} = 3.6 \text{ ml/hour}$$

Answer: The rate required $= 3.6$ ml/hour.

G.19 (i) Beware of units. Convert 5 mg to micrograms ($= 5,000$ mcg).

Answer: The rate is 30 ml/hour.

(ii) 10 drops/min – SGS (20 drops/ml)
30 drops/min – microdrop giving set (60 drops/ml)

G.20 (i) Beware of units. Convert 50 mg to micrograms ($= 50,000$ mcg).

Dose required $= 2$ mcg/kg/min   Weight $= 60$ kg
$= 2 \times 60 = 120$ mcg/min

Answer: The rate is 14.4 ml/hour (14 ml/hour).

(ii) 4.8 drops/min (5 drops/min) – SGS (20 drops/ml)
14.4 drops/min (14 drops/min) – micro-drop giving set (60 drops/ml)

G.21 (i) Beware of units. Convert 50 mg to micrograms ($= 50,000$ mcg).
Answer: The rate is 90 ml/hour.

(ii) 30 drops/min – SGS (20 drops/ml)
90 drops/min – microdrop giving set (60 drops/ml)

G.22 (i) 90 ml/hour
(ii) 30 drops/min – SGS (20 drops/ml)
90 drops/min – microdrop giving set (60 drops/ml)

G.23 (i) You have 5 mg in 500 ml. Calculate the number of milligrams in 1 ml by dividing by 500:

$$\frac{5}{500} = \frac{1}{100} \text{ mg in 1 ml}$$

Convert milligrams to micrograms by multiplying by 1,000:

$$\frac{1}{100} \times 1,000 = 10 \text{ mcg/ml}$$

Answer: 10 mcg/ml

(ii) Beware of units. Convert 5 mg to micrograms
(= 5,000 mcg).
Answer: The rate is 30 ml/hour.

(iii) 10 drops/min – SGS (20 drops/ml)
30 drops/min – microdrop giving set (60 drops/ml)

G.24 (i) Dose required = Dose (5 mcg/kg/min) × Patient's
weight (73 kg)
= 5 × 73 = 365 mcg/min

(ii) Beware of units. Convert 250 mg to micrograms
(= 250,000 mcg). Therefore you have 250,000 mcg in
500 ml. To find the concentration (mcg/ml), divide by
500:

$$\frac{250,000}{500} = 500$$

Answer: 500 mcg/ml

(iii) 43.8 ml/hour (44 ml/hour)

(iv) 14.6 drops/min (15 drops/min) – SGS (20 drops/ml)
43.8 drops/min (44 drops/min) – microdrop giving set
(60 drops/ml)

G.25 (i) The rate = 2 mg/hour. Convert mg to ml. You have
50 mg in 500 ml. Therefore:

$$1 \, mg = \frac{500}{50} = 10 \, ml$$

Thus:

$$2 \, mg/hour = 10 \times 2 = 20 \, ml/hour$$

Answer: The rate = 20 ml/hour.

(ii) First convert the rate from mg/hour to mg/min. Rate
required = 2 mg/hour, which is equal to:

$$\frac{2}{60} = \frac{1}{30} \, mg/min$$

Now you have to convert the 'dose in mg' to a 'dose in ml'. You have an infusion of 50 mg in 500 ml. Therefore calculate the volume for 1 mg:

$$1\,\text{mg} = \frac{500}{50} = 10\,\text{ml}$$

However, the rate required is $\frac{1}{30}$ mg, which equals:

$$\frac{1}{30} \times 10 = \frac{1}{3}\,\text{ml/min}$$

(the dose is converted to a volume). Now you have to convert this volume to drops by multiplying by the drip rate for the giving set being used. If using a standard giving set (20 drop/ml):

$$\frac{1}{3} \times 20 = 6.67\,\text{drops/min}\;(7\,\text{drops/min})$$

If using a micro-drop giving set (60 drops/ml):

$$\frac{1}{3} \times 60 = 20\,\text{drops/min}$$

Answer: 6.67 drops/min (7 drops/min) – SGS
(20 drops/ml)
20 drops/min – microdrop giving set
(60 drops/ml)

If using the formula:

$$\text{Drops/min} = \frac{\text{Total volume to be infused}}{\text{Total amount of drug}} \times \text{Dose} \times \text{Drip rate of giving set}$$

where:

Total volume to be infused $= 500\,\text{ml}$
Total amount of drug (mg) $= 50\,\text{mg}$
Dose $= 1/30\,\text{mg}$ (as worked out previously)
Drip rate of the giving set $= 20\,\text{drops/ml}$

substitute the numbers in the formula:

$$\frac{500}{50} \times \frac{1}{30} \times 20 = 6.67 \text{ drops/min (7 drops/min)}$$

Answer: 6.67 drops/min (7 drops/min) – SGS (20 drops/ml)
20 drops/min – microdrop giving set (60 drops/ml)

(iii) *Answer:* The rate = 50 ml/hour.

(iv) Convert the new rate from mg/hour to mg/min. Rate required = 5 mg/hour, which is equal to:

$$\frac{5}{60} = \frac{1}{12} \text{mg/min}$$

Now calculate the new rate as before.

Answer: 16.6 drops/min (17 drops/min) – SGS (20 drops/ml)
50 drops/min – microdrop giving set (60 drops/ml)

Conversion of ml/hour to dosages

G.26 Convert the amount of drug to micrograms (same units):

200 mg = 200 × 1,000 = 200,000 mcg

Therefore you have 200,000 mcg in 50 ml. Thus in 1 ml, you have:

$$\frac{200,000}{50} \text{mcg}$$

The rate at which the pump is running is 4 ml/hour. You have just worked out the amount of dopamine in 1 ml, therefore in 4 ml:

$$\frac{200,000}{50} \times 4 \text{mcg/hour}$$

To convert the rate to mcg/min, divide by 60:

$$\frac{200{,}000}{50 \times 60} \times 4 \text{ mcg/min}$$

To find out the rate in terms of the patient's weight, divide by the patient's weight (89 kg):

$$\frac{200{,}000 \times 4}{50 \times 60 \times 89} = 2.99 \text{ mcg/kg/min (3 mcg/kg/min)}$$

Answer: The dose is correct. No adjustment is necessary.

If using the formula:

$$\text{mcg/kg/min} = \frac{\text{Rate (ml/hour)} \times \text{Amount of drug (mcg)}}{60 \times \text{Weight (kg)} \times \text{Volume (ml)}}$$

where:

Rate	= 4 ml/hour
Amount of drug (mcg)	= 200,000 mcg
Weight (kg)	= 89 kg
Volume (ml)	= 50 ml

substitute the numbers in the formula:

$$\frac{4 \times 200{,}000}{60 \times 89 \times 50} = 2.99 \text{ mcg/kg/min (3 mcg/kg/min)}$$

Answer: The dose is correct. No adjustment is necessary.

G.27 Convert the amount of drug to micrograms (same units):

$$250 \text{ mg} = 250 \times 1{,}000 = 250{,}000 \text{ mcg}$$

Therefore you have 250,000 mcg in 50 ml, thus in 1 ml you have:

$$\frac{250{,}000}{50} \text{ mcg}$$

The rate at which the pump is running is 5.6 ml/hour. You have just worked out the amount in 1 ml. So in 5.6 ml:

$$\frac{250{,}000}{50} \times 5.6 \text{ mcg/hour}$$

To convert the rate to mcg/min, divide by 60:

$$\frac{250,000}{50 \times 60} \times 5.6 \, \text{mcg/min}$$

To find out the rate in terms of the patient's weight, divide by the patient's weight (64 kg):

$$\frac{250,000 \times 5.6}{50 \times 60 \times 64} = 7.29 \, \text{mcg/kg/min} \, (7 \, \text{mcg/kg/min})$$

Answer: 7.29 mcg/kg/min (7 mcg/kg/min, 'rounded down')

The dose being delivered by the pump set at a rate of 5.6 ml/hour is too high. Inform the doctor and adjust the rate of the pump.

If using the formula:

$$\text{mcg/kg/min} = \frac{\text{Rate (ml/hour)} \times \text{Amount of drug (mcg)}}{60 \times \text{Weight (kg)} \times \text{Volume (ml)}}$$

where:

Rate	= 5.6 ml/hour
Amount of drug (mcg)	= 250,000 mcg
Weight (kg)	= 64 kg
Volume (ml)	= 50 ml

substitute the numbers in the formula:

$$\frac{5.6 \times 250,000}{60 \times 64 \times 50} = 7.29 \, \text{mcg/kg/min} \, (7 \, \text{mcg/kg/min})$$

Answer: 7.29 mcg/kg/min (7 mcg/kg/min, 'rounded down')

The dose being delivered by the pump set at a rate of 5.6 ml/hour is too high. Inform the doctor and adjust the rate of the pump.

Changing the rate of the pump

In this case, the calculation is done the other way round, starting at the dose. The dose required is 6 mcg/kg/min. The patient's weight is 64 kg, therefore the dose for the patient equals:

$$6 \times 64 = 384 \text{ mcg/min}$$

To find the dose per hour, multiply by 60:

$$384 \times 60 = 23{,}040 \text{ mcg/hour}$$

You have 50/250,000 ml/mcg of dobutamine (worked out previously). Therefore to find the volume per hour for the dose, multiply by 23,040:

$$\frac{50}{250{,}000} \times 23{,}040 = 4.608 \text{ ml/hour} \ (4.6 \text{ ml/hour})$$

Answer: The rate at which the pump should have been set equals 4.6 ml/hour and not 5.6 ml/hour.

Alternatively, use the formula:

$$\text{mcg/kg/min} = \frac{\text{Rate (ml/hour)} \times \text{Amount of drug (mcg)}}{60 \times \text{Weight (kg)} \times \text{Volume (ml)}}$$

In this case, the unknown is the rate (ml/hour). So the formula needs to be rewritten:

$$\text{Rate (ml/hour)} = \frac{\text{Dose (mcg/kg/min)} \times \text{Weight (kg)} \times \text{Volume (ml)} \times 60}{\text{Amount of drug (mcg)}}$$

where:

Dose (mcg/kg/min)	= 6 mcg/kg/min
Weight (kg)	= 64 kg
Volume (ml)	= 50 ml
Amount of drug (mcg)	= 250,000 mcg

Substitute the numbers in the formula:

$$\frac{6 \times 64 \times 50 \times 60}{250{,}000} = 4.6 \text{ ml/hour}$$

Answer: The rate at which the pump should have been set equals 4.6 ml/hour and not 5.6 ml/hour.

G.28 The dose on the prescription chart = 0.5 mcg/kg/min.

Answer: The dose is correct. No adjustment is necessary.

G.29 You have 250 mg frusemide in 100 ml. First, work out the amount of frusemide in 1 ml:

250 mg in 100 ml

$\dfrac{250}{100}$ mg in 1 ml

The pump is delivering at a rate of 50 ml/hour, so work out the amount of frusemide the pump is delivering per hour:

$$\frac{250}{100} \times 50 = 125 \text{ mg}$$

So the pump is delivering 125 mg per hour. Next, divide by 60 to find the amount per minute:

$$\frac{125}{60} = 2.08 \text{ mg/min } (2 \text{ mg/min})$$

Answer: The pump is delivering frusemide at a rate of 2 mg/min, which is within the recommended rate of 4 mg/min.

If using the formula:

$$\text{mg/min} = \frac{\text{Rate (ml/hour)} \times \text{Amount of drug (mg)}}{60 \times \text{Volume (ml)}}$$

where:

Rate = 50 ml/hour
Amount of drug (mcg) = 250 mg
Volume (ml) = 100 ml

substitute the numbers in the formula:

$$\frac{50 \times 250}{60 \times 100} = 2.08 \text{ mg/min } (2 \text{ mg/min})$$

Answer: The pump is delivering frusemide at a rate of 2 mg/min, which is within the recommended rate of 4 mg/min.

G.30 The pump is delivering at a rate of 3 mg/min, which is the same as the prescribed dose.

G.31 Convert the amount of isoprenaline to micrograms (the dose is in micrograms):

Isoprenaline 2 mg = 2 × 1,000 = 2,000 mcg

Now calculate the rate as before.

Answer: The pump is delivering at a rate of 3 mcg/min, which is the same as the prescribed dose.

Calculating the length of time for I.V. infusions

G.32 First, convert the volume to drops by multiplying the volume of the infusion by the number of drops/ml for the giving set:

1,000 × 20 = 20,000 drops

Next, calculate how many minutes it will take for 1 drop, i.e.

21 drops per minute

1 drop in $\frac{1}{21}$ mins

Calculate how many minutes it will take to infuse the total number of drops:

20,000 drops in $\frac{1}{21}$ × 20,000 = 952 min

Convert minutes to hours by dividing by 60:

952 min = $\frac{952}{60}$ = 15.87 hours

15.87 hours = 15 hours 52 min (approx. 16 hours)

Answer: 1 litre of sodium chloride at a rate of 21 drops/min will take approximately 16 hours to run.

If using the formula:

$$\text{Number of hours the infusion is to run} = \frac{\text{Volume of the infusion}}{\text{Rate (drop/min)} \times 60} \times \text{Drip rate of giving set}$$

where:

Volume of the infusion = 1,000 ml
Rate (drops/min) = 21 drops/min
Drip rate of giving set = 20 drops/ml

substitute the numbers in the formula:

$$\frac{1,000}{21 \times 60} \times 20 = 15.87 \text{ hours}$$

15.87 hours = 15 hours 52 min (approx. 16 hours)

Answer: 1 litre of sodium chloride at a rate of 21 drops/min will take approximately 16 hours to run.

G.33 66.67 minutes (67 minutes, approx.)

G.34 4.17 hours (4 hours, 10 minutes), approx. 4 hours

G.35 (i) 8.33 hours (8 hours, 20 minutes), approx. 8 hours

(ii) First, calculate what volume has already been infused (4 hours at 20 drops/min). Convert hours to minutes:

4 hours = 4 × 60 = 240 minutes

Now calculate the volume that has already been infused by multiplying the rate by the number of minutes:

20 × 240 = 4,800 drops

Calculate the volume infused (in ml) by dividing the number of drops by the drip rate of the giving set (20 drops/ml):

$$\frac{4,800}{20} = 240 \text{ ml}$$

Thus after 4 hours, 240 ml of the infusion has already been infused. Therefore, there are $500 - 240 = 260$ ml left. Now calculate how long it would take to infuse 260 ml at the new rate of 30 drops/min.

Answer: 2.89 hours (2 hours, 53 minutes), approx. 3 hours

G.36 (i) Rate should be 4 mg/min or 1 mg over $\frac{1}{4}$ min. Amount of drug being infused = 250 mg. Therefore the time for 250 mg should be:

$$\frac{1}{4} \times 250 = 62.5 \, \text{min}$$

So the infusion should take no less than an hour.

(ii) Convert the volume being infused to drops by multiplying the volume by the number of drops per ml for the giving set:

$$100 \, \text{ml} = 100 \times 20 = 2{,}000 \, \text{drops (using a SGS)}$$

From the rate (42 drops/min), calculate how long it would take for 1 drop, i.e.

42 drops in 1 min

1 drop in $\frac{1}{42}$ min

However, you want to know how long it would take to infuse 2,000 drops. So multiply the time for 1 drop by the total number of drops, i.e.

$$\frac{1}{42} \times 2{,}000 = 47.7 \, \text{min} \, (48 \, \text{min})$$

If using the formula:

$$\text{Number of minutes the infusion is to run} = \frac{\text{Volume of the infusion}}{\text{Rate (drops/min)}} \times \text{Drip rate of giving set}$$

where:

Volume of the infusion = 100 ml
Rate (drops/min)   = 42 drops/min
Drip rate of giving set = 20 drops/ml

substitute the numbers in the formula:

$$\frac{100}{42} \times 20 = 47.7 \text{ min } (48 \text{ min})$$

So the rate is too fast. The infusion should be stopped
and a new rate calculated.

The rate should be 4 mg/min, and this has to be
converted to drops/min to give the new rate. The
concentration of frusemide is 250 mg in 100 ml. This is
equal to:

$$\frac{250}{100} = 2.5 \text{ mg/ml (or } 1 \text{ mg } = 1/2.5 \text{ ml)}$$

Thus 4 mg/min is equal to $\frac{4}{2.5}$ ml/min.

The next step is to convert this to drops/min. The
number of drops per ml for the giving set = 20
drops/ml (SGS) So:

$$\frac{4}{2.5} \text{ ml/min} = \frac{4}{2.5} \times 20 = 32 \text{ drops/min}$$

The proper infusion rate is 32 drops/min and *not* 42
drops/min.

G.37 (i) Maximum rate should be 10 mg/min or 1 mg over
$\frac{1}{10}$ min. Amount of drug being infused = 1 g or
1,000 mg. Therefore the time for 1,000 mg should be:

$$\frac{1}{10} \times 1,000 = 100 \text{ min}$$

The minimum time over which the infusion can be
given is 100 minutes. So give the infusion over 2 hours.

(ii) Convert the volume being infused to drops by multiplying
the volume by the number of drops per ml for the
giving set:

$$200\,\text{ml} = 200 \times 20 = 4{,}000 \text{ drops (using a SGS)}$$

From the rate (50 drops/min), calculate how long it would take for 1 drop, i.e.

50 drops in 1 min

$$1 \text{ drop in } \frac{1}{50}\,\text{min}$$

However, you want to know how long it would take to infuse 4,000 drops. So multiply the time for 1 drop by the total number of drops, i.e.

$$\frac{1}{50} \times 4{,}000 = 80\,\text{min}$$

If using the formula:

$$\text{Number of minutes the infusion is to run} = \frac{\text{Volume of the infusion}}{\text{Rate (drops/min)}} \times \text{Drip rate of giving set}$$

where:

Volume of the infusion = 200 ml
Rate (drops/min) = 50 drops/min
Drip rate of giving set = 20 drops/ml

substitute the numbers in the formula:

$$\frac{200}{50} \times 20 = 80\,\text{min}$$

So the rate is too fast. The infusion should be stopped and a new rate calculated.

The rate should be 10 mg/min, and this has to be converted to drops/min to give the new rate. The concentration of vancomycin is 1,000 mg in 200 ml. This is equal to

$$\frac{1{,}000}{200} = 5\,\text{mg/ml}$$

Thus 10 mg/min is equal to 2 ml/min.

The next step is to convert this to drops/min. The number of drops per ml for the giving set = 20 drops/ml (SGS). So:

2 ml/min = 2 × 20 = 40 drops/min

The proper infusion rate is 40 drops/min and *not* 50 drops/min.

10 *Paediatric dosage calculations*

··

OBJECTIVES
At the end of this section you should be familiar with the following:
Different methods of calculation
  Body weight calculations
  Body surface area estimates
  Percentage method

Problems associated with paediatric doses
Displacement values for injections
Routes of administration
  Oral administration
  Intravenous administration (infusions)

INTRODUCTION

When it comes to prescribing and administering medicines to children, they shouldn't be considered as small adults and care should be taken in calculating doses.

This is because all children, and particularly neonates, differ in their response to drugs, i.e. absorption, distribution, metabolism of a drug, and its effects and duration of action.

METHOD OF CALCULATION

Children's doses may be calculated from adult doses by using age, body weight, or body surface area, or by a combination of all these factors. Many formulae have been devised (e.g. Clark's rule and Young's rule), but they are not accurate for all children.

Doses related to age are not sufficiently accurate to compensate for the great variability in weights. Dosage calculations based on weights are better, but not ideal.

With most drugs, adults and older children receive too much drug if given infant doses on a 'mg/kg' basis. Conversely, infants may receive too little drug if they are given mg/kg doses for adults and large children. This is due to the fact that hepatic metabolism in the neonate and infant is faster for some drugs (compared to older children and adults), since they have a greater liver volume per unit body weight. Consequently neonates and infants will need a higher mg/kg dose to overcome this faster rate of metabolism.

Using body surface area is the most accurate method, but even this fails to take into account the differences between children and adults in some parameters and tissue responsiveness.

However, as clinical knowledge and experience has increased, there are specialist paediatric books now available that give

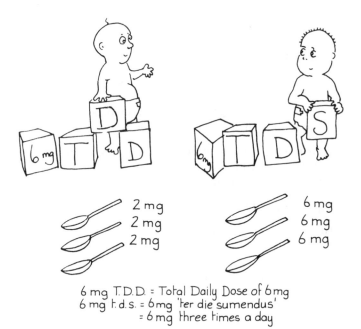

6 mg T.D.D. = Total Daily Dose of 6mg
6 mg t.d.s. = 6mg 'ter die sumendus'
= 6mg three times a day

accurate doses on a 'dose per weight' basis (mg/kg) and these should be consulted first (a list appears at the end of this section).

CALCULATING DOSAGES

When doing any calculation, you must *make sure that the decimal point is in the right place*. A change to the left or right would mean a 10-fold change in the dose which could be fatal in some cases.

It is best to work in the smaller units, i.e. 100 micrograms as opposed to 0.1 milligrams. But even so, care must be taken with the number of noughts; a wrong dose can be fatal.

When calculating any dose – always get your answer checked

Body weight calculations

This is the most common method for calculating paediatric dosages.

When reading doses for paediatrics, it is important that they are interpreted correctly. They can be written as either:

(a) a single dose – to be given as many times as specified, or
(b) total daily dose (T.D.D.) – to be divided by the number of times the drug is to be given.

For example, oral salbutamol can be written as:

100 mcg/kg, 4 times a day

or

400 mcg/kg/day (400 mcg/kg T.D.D.)

Care must be taken that a total daily dose is not mistaken for a single dose.

WORKED EXAMPLE

Salbutamol is to be administered to a 3-year-old child weighing 13.5 kg at a dose of 100 mcg/kg four times a day.

Therefore, you simply multiply the dose by the weight, i.e. in this case:

$100 \times 13.5 = 1{,}350 \, mcg$

What you have is a bottle containing salbutamol 2 mg in 5 ml, therefore you have to convert your dose from micrograms to milligrams (divide by 1,000):

$$1{,}350 \, mcg = \frac{1{,}350}{1{,}000} = 1.35 \, mg = 1.4 \, mg \, (\text{'rounding up'})$$

Therefore the dose you need to give is 1.4 mg four times a day.

However, as already stated, you have salbutamol liquid 2 mg in 5 ml. Therefore you now need to calculate how much you need for your dose of 1.4 mg. You have 2 mg in 5 ml. Therefore:

$$1 \, mg \, in \, \frac{5}{2} \, ml$$

(using the '**one** unit' rule). But you need 1.4 mg, which equals:

$$\frac{5}{2} \times 1.4 = 3.5 \, ml$$

Therefore you need to give 3.5 ml of the salbutamol liquid (2 mg in 5 ml) four times day.

For a more detailed explanation of this method of calculation, see Section 4 on Dosage calculations.

When using this method of calculation, the actual body weight should be used. However, in the case of obese children, the child may receive an artificially high dose. The reason for this is that fat tissue plays virtually no part in metabolism, and the dose must be estimated on lean or ideal body weight.

However, as a rule of thumb, the dose should be reduced by approximately 25% for the obese child.

Similarly, the dose should be adjusted if the child has oedema, or is dehydrated, or is pyrexial.

As stated before, many formulae have been devised to calculate dosages, but are now regarded as inaccurate and, perhaps, obsolete.

One example is based on Clark's rule, giving a mg/kg dose:

$$\frac{\text{Adult dose (in kg)}}{70 \text{ kg}} = \text{mg/kg dose}$$

where 70 kg is the weight of an average adult male.

Thus in the above example of salbutamol, the mg/kg dose, using this formula, would be:

Adult dose of oral salbutamol $= 4 \text{ mg}$

$$\frac{4}{70} = 0.057 \text{ mg/kg} = 57 \text{ mcg/kg}$$

Thus for a 3-year-old child weighing 13.5 kg, using this formula, the total dose $= 57 \times 13.5 = 769.5 \text{ mcg}$ (0.8 mg).

As you can see, there is a wide difference in dose using the two methods. This can be important if the drug concerned has a narrow therapeutic range, i.e. a small difference exists between the therapeutic and toxic doses.

Similarly, dosage may be expressed in terms of body surface area (mg/m^2). The dose required is calculated in the same way, but substituting surface area for weight. In this case, the surface area needs to be worked out by using either tables or nomograms (see Appendix 1 on how to use nomograms).

Body surface area (B.S.A.) estimates

This is a more accurate method than formulae using body weight, since many physical phenomena are more closely related to body surface area.

The average body surface area of a 70 kg person is about 1.8 m^2.

Thus to calculate the dose for a child, the following formula may be used:

$$\frac{\text{Surface area of child (m}^2)}{1.8} \times \text{Adult dose}$$

Once again, surface areas can be calculated from nomograms or from tables. In the original example of salbutamol:

$$\frac{0.62}{1.8} \times 4 = 1.38\,\text{mg} = 1.4\,\text{mg} \text{ ('rounding up')}$$

where the surface area for a 3-year-old child $= 0.62\,\text{m}^2$.

As you can see, the dose is the same as using a paediatric dosage book, so this method can be considered quite accurate.

Percentage method

In this method, the dose is calculated as a percentage of the adult dose. It should only be used for drugs that have a wide margin between the therapeutic and the toxic dose.

The percentage is either given in tables (see Table 10.2 later in this section), or calculated using a formula.

Once again, using our original example of salbutamol, the percentage of the adult dose needed is 33%. The adult dose = 4 mg, therefore:

$$33\% = \frac{4}{100} \times 33 = 1.32\,\text{mg} = 1.3\,\text{mg} \text{ ('rounding down')}$$

Or it can be calculated by using the formula:

$$\frac{\text{Surface area of child } (\text{m}^2)}{1.8} \times 100 = \% \text{ of adult dose}$$

In the present case the surface area for a 3-year-old child = $0.62\,\text{m}^2$, therefore:

$$\frac{0.62}{1.8} \times 100 = 34.4\% = 34\% \text{ ('rounding down')}$$

Therefore the dose for the 3-year-old child using this method would be:

$$\frac{4}{100} \times 34 = 1.36\,\text{mg} = 1.4\,\text{mg} \text{ ('rounding up')}$$

Thus, there are several methods available for calculating paediatric dosages. Table 10.1 compares the answers obtained by these methods.

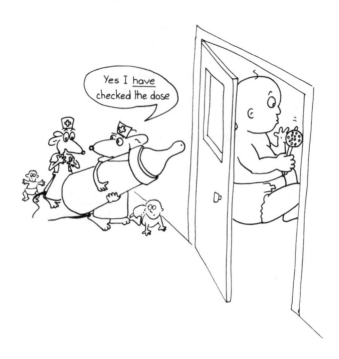

As you can see from Table 10.1, apart from the body weight estimates, all the other methods give approximately the same answer. However, there are a few reservations when using formulae for calculating dosages.

TABLE 10.1 Dose of oral salbutamol for a 3-year-old child using different methods of calculation

Method	Dose
From a paediatric reference book	1.35 mg (1.4 mg)
Body weight estimate from an adult dose	0.8 mg
Body surface area estimates	1.38 mg (1.4 mg)
Percentage methods (see text example)	(i) 1.32 mg (1.3 mg)
	(ii) 1.36 mg (1.4 mg)

(a) They should only be used for drugs which have a wide margin between the therapeutic and toxic dose, i.e. have a wide margin of safety.

(b) When using methods of calculation based on adult doses, there may be more than one dose to choose from. For example, from the British National Formulary (B.N.F.), the dose quoted for the adult oral dose of salbutamol can be 4 mg or 8 mg. Thus either of two doses can be used. In the example the 4 mg dose was used, but if the higher 8 mg dose were used then the answer, obviously, would be double.

> Therefore doses should be calculated from specialist paediatric books, and not from general formulae. These should only be used if a specific dose is not found, or to check a dose.

PROBLEMS ASSOCIATED WITH PAEDIATRIC DOSE CALCULATIONS

As stated before, doses may have to be adjusted for the following:

1. Renal or hepatic insufficiency
2. Fever
3. Oedema
4. Dehydration
5. Gastrointestinal (G.I.) disease

In these cases, the doctor should decide whether a dose needs to be adjusted.

Whatever the method of calculation used, there will be occasions when it will be difficult to give the dose required due to the lack of an appropriate formulation, for example to give 33 mg when only a 100 mg tablet is available. In these instances, it is advisable that the pharmacy department should be contacted to see if a liquid preparation is available or can be prepared. If not, the doctor should be informed so that the dose can be modified, or another drug can be prescribed, or another route can be used.

Table 10.2 lists approximate average values of various parameters, but this method of calculating doses should only be used

TABLE 10.2 Average values for various parameters useful in calculating children's doses

Age	Weight		Height		Surface area m^2	% of adult dose
	kg	lb	cm	in		
Newborn	3.4	7.5	50	20	0.23	12.5
1 month	4.2	9	55	22	0.26	14.5
2 months	4.5	10	52	21	0.28	15.0
3 months	5.6	12	59	23	0.32	18.0
4 months	6.5	14	62	24	0.36	20.0
6 months	7.7	17	67	26	0.40	22.0
8 months	8.5	19	72	28	0.44	25.0
1 year	10	22	76	30	0.47	28.0
18 months	11	24	90	35	0.53	30.0
3 years	14	31	94	37	0.62	33.0
5 years	18	40	108	42	0.73	40.0
7 years	23	51	120	47	0.88	50.0
10 years	30	66	142	56	1.09	60.0
12 years	37	81	145	58	1.25	75.0
14 years	45	110	150	59	1.38	80.0
16 years	58	128	167	67	1.65	90.0
Adult male	68	150	173	68	1.80	
Adult female	56	123	163	64	1.60	

if a specific dose cannot be found, since it assumes the child is 'average'.

DISPLACEMENT VALUES OR VOLUMES

Displacement values or volumes are usually given to freeze-dried injections, particularly antibiotics, that need to be reconstituted before administration.

This is the volume of fluid displaced by the powder and must be taken into account where part vials are being used. If this is not done, significant errors in dosage may occur, especially when small doses are involved as with neonates.

Displacement volumes are usually stated in the relevant data sheets, or in paediatric dosage books.

EXAMPLE

Cefotaxime at a dose of 50 mg/kg, 12 hourly for a baby weighing 3.6 kg. Therefore the dose required equals:

$$50 \times 3.6 = 180 \, mg$$

Displacement volume for cefotaxime = 0.2 ml for a 500 mg vial. Therefore you need to add 1.8 ml water for injection to give:

500 mg in 2 ml

Thus 180 mg in 0.72 ml.

If the displacement volume is not taken into account, then you will have:

500 mg in 2.2 ml (2 ml + 0.2 ml displacement volume)

You worked out earlier that 180 mg = 0.72 ml (assuming 500 mg in 2 ml). But in this case, 0.72 ml equals:

$$\frac{500}{2.2} \times 0.72 = 164 \, mg$$

Thus if the displacement volume is not taken into account, then the amount drawn up is 164 mg and not 180 mg as expected.

Some useful approximations

The following are only approximate values and should not be taken as true values:

1. Weight in kg = (Age in years + 3) × 2.5
2. Surface area in $m^2 = \dfrac{(\text{Age in years} + 6) \times 7}{100}$
3. Percentage of adult dose = (Weight in kg × 1.5) + 10
4. Percentage of adult dose = (Age in years × 4) + 20 (more accurate than the formula in 3)

TABLE 10.3 Displacement volumes for various injections

Drug	Displacement volume	Reconstitute with	Final volume	Dosage guide
Cardiovascular system				
ALTEPLASE 50mg (Actilyse, Boehringer)	Zero	50ml water	50ml	1mg in 1ml
ANISTREPLASE 30 units (Eminase, SB)	0.1ml/30 units	4.9ml water	5ml	6 units in 1ml
EPOPROSTENOL 500μg (Flolan, Wellcome)	Negligible	50ml diluent	50ml	10μg in 1ml
HYDRALAZINE 20mg (Apresoline, Ciba)	0.14ml/20mg	0.86ml water	1ml	20mg in 1ml
SODIUM NITROPRUSSIDE 50mg (Nipride, Roche)	Negligible	2ml diluent	2ml	25mg in 1ml
STREPTOKINASE 1,500,000 units (Streptase, Hoechst)	Zero	50ml sodium chloride	50ml	30,000 units in 1ml
UROKINASE 5,000 units (Leo)	Zero	2ml water	2ml	2,500 units in 1ml
Central nervous system				
AMYLOBARBITONE SODIUM 500mg (Sodium Amytal, Lily)	0.33ml/500mg	49.67ml water	50ml	For a 1% solution
		4.67ml water	5ml	For a 10% solution
BOTULINUM TOXIN 500 units (Dysport, Porton)	Zero	2.5ml water	2.5ml	200 units in 1ml
DIAMORPHINE 5mg (Napp)	0.06m/5mg	0.94ml water	1ml	5mg in 1ml
SODIUM VALPROATE 400mg (Epilim I/V, Sanofi)	0.35ml/400mg	3.65ml diluent	4ml	100mg in 1ml
Infections				
ACYCLOVIR 250mg (Zovirax, Wellcome)	Negligible	10ml water	10ml	25mg in 1ml
AMOXYCILLIN 250mg (Amoxil, Bencard)	0.2ml/250mg	1.8ml water	2ml	125mg in 1ml
AMPHOTERICIN 50mg (Fungizone, Squibb)	Negligible	10ml water	10ml	5mg in 1ml
AMPHOTERICIN LIPOSOMAL 50mg (Ambisome, Vestar)	0.5ml/50mg	12ml water	12.5ml	4mg in 1ml
AMPICILLIN 250mg (Penbrittin, Beecham)	0.2ml/250mg	1.8ml water	2ml	125mg in 1ml
AMPICLOX (Beecham)	0.4ml/500mg	1.6ml water	2ml	250mg in 1ml
AZLOCILLIN 500mg (Securopen, Bayer)	0.37ml/500mg	4.63ml water	5ml	100mg in 1ml

TABLE 10.3 (contd)

Drug	Displacement volume	Reconstitute with	Final volume	Dosage guide
AZTREONAM 500mg (Azactam, Squibb)	0.4ml/500mg	3.6ml water	4ml	125mg in 1ml
BENZYLPENICILLIN 600mg (Crystapen, Brittania)	0.4ml/600mg	1.6ml water	2ml	300mg in 1ml
CAPREOMYCIN 1g (Capastat, Dista)	0.7ml/gram	2.3ml water	3ml	300mg in 0.9ml
CARBENICILLIN 1g (Pyopen, Goldshield)	0.75ml/gram	3.25ml water	4ml	250mg in 1ml
CEFODIZIME 1g (Timecef, Roussel)	0.56ml/gram	3.44ml water	4ml	250mg in 1ml
CEFOTAXIME 500mg (Claforan, Roussel)	0.2ml/500mg	1.8ml water	2ml	250mg in 1ml
CEFOXITIN 1g (Mefoxin, MSD)	0.5ml/gram	2ml water	2.5ml	400mg in 1ml
CEFSULODIN 1g (Monaspor, Ciba)	0.65ml/gram	3.35ml water	4ml	250mg in 1ml
CEFTAZIDIME 500mg (Fortum, Glaxo)	0.55ml/500mg	1.45ml water	2ml	250mg in 1ml
CEFTIZOXIME 500mg (Cefizox, Wellcome)	0.3ml/500mg	2.2ml water	2.5ml	200mg in 1ml
CEFTRIAXONE 250mg (Rocephin, Roche)	0.19ml/250mg	4.81ml water	5ml	50mg in 1ml
CEFUROXIME 250mg (Zinacef, Glaxo)	0.18ml/250mg	1.82ml water	2ml	125mg in 1ml
CEPHAMANDOLE 500mg (Kefadol, Dista)	0.35ml/500mg	1.15ml water	1.5ml	250mg in 0.75ml
CEPHAZOLIN 500mg (Kefzol, Dista)	0.3ml/500mg	2.2ml water	2.5ml	200mg in 1ml
CEPHRADINE 500mg (Velosef, Squibb)	0.4ml/500mg	2.1ml water	2.5ml	200mg in 1ml
CHLORAMPHENICOL 300mg (Chloromycetin, Parke Davis)	0.25ml/300mg	11.75ml water	12ml	25mg in 1ml
CHLORAMPHENICOL 1g (Kemicetine, Farmitalia)	0.8ml/gram	9.2ml water	10ml	100mg in 1ml
CHLORAMPHENICOL 1.2g (Chloromycetin, Parke Davis)	1ml/1.2g	11ml water	12ml	100mg in 1ml
CLOXACILLIN 250mg (Orbenin, Beecham)	0.2ml/250mg	1.8ml water	2ml	125mg in 1ml
CO-AMOXICLAV 600mg (Augmentin, Beecham)	0.5ml/600mg	9.5ml water	10ml	60mg in 1ml
CO-FLUAMPICIL 500mg (Magnapen, Beecham)	0.4ml/500mg	1.6ml water	2ml	250mg in 1ml

TABLE 10.3 (contd)

Drug	Displacement volume	Reconstitute with	Final volume	Dosage guide
COLISTIN 1 megaunit (Colomycin, Pharmax)	0.02ml/million units	1.98ml water	2ml	500,000 units in 1ml
ERYTHROMYCIN 1g (Abbott)	Allowed for	20ml water	22ml	Contains 1g in 20ml 50mg in 1ml
FLUCLOXACILLIN 250mg (Floxapen, Beecham)	0.2ml/250mg	1.8ml water	2ml	125mg in 1ml
FUSIDATE SODIUM 500mg (Fucidin, Leo)	Negligible	10ml buffer	10ml	50mg in 1ml
GANCICLOVIR 500mg (Cymevene, Syntex)	0.29ml/500mg	9.71ml water	10ml	50mg in 1ml
IMIPENEM/CILASTATIN 250mg (Primaxin, MSD)	Negligible	50ml water	50ml	5mg in 1ml
KANAMYCIN 1g (Kannasyn, Sanofi Winthrop)	0.8ml/g	4.2ml water	5ml	200mg in 1ml
MECILLINAM 400mg (Selexidin, Leo)	0.1ml/400mg	1.9ml water	2ml	200mg in 1ml
METHICILLIN 1g (Celbenin, Goldshield)	0.7ml/g	1.8ml water	2.5ml	400mg in 1ml
PENTAMIDINE 300mg (Pentacarinat, RPR)	0.15ml/300mg	3.85ml water	4ml	75mg in 1ml
PIPERACILLIN 1g (Pipril, Lederle)	0.73ml/g	3.27ml water	4ml	250mg in 1ml
POLYMYXIN B SULPHATE 500,000 units (Aerosporin, Wellcome)	Zero	1ml water	1ml	500,000 units in 1ml
PROCAINE PENICILLIN 3 megaunits (Bicillin, Brocades)	1.4ml/vial	4.6ml water	6ml	500,000 units in 1ml
RIFAMPICIN 300mg (Rifadin, Merrell; Rimactane, Ciba)	0.24ml/300mg	4.76ml solvent	5ml	60mg in 1ml
SPECTINOMYCIN 2g (Trobicin, Upjohn)	1.8ml/2g	3.2ml diluent	5ml	400mg in 1ml
STREPTOMYCIN 1g (Evans)	0.75ml/g	1.25ml water	2ml	500mg in 1ml
TAZOCIN 2.25g (Lederle)	0.7ml/g	13.4ml water	15ml	150mg in 1ml
TEICOPLANIN 200mg (Targocid, Merrell)	Allowed for	3ml diluent	3ml	50mg in 0.75ml
TEMOCILLIN 500mg (Temopen, Bencard)	0.35ml/500mg	1.65ml water	2ml	250mg in 1ml

TABLE 10.3 (contd)

Drug	Displacement volume	Reconstitute with	Final volume	Dosage guide
TETRACYCLINE 100mg (Achromycin, Lederle)	0.3ml/100mg	2.2ml water	2.5ml	40mg in 1ml
TETRACYCLINE 250mg (Achromycin I/V, Lederle)	0.15ml/250mg	4.85ml water	5ml	50mg in 1ml
TICARCILLIN 1g (Ticar, Goldshield)	0.7ml/g	3.3ml water	4ml	250mg in 1ml
TIMENTIN 800mg (Beecham)	0.55ml/800mg	4.45ml water	5ml	160mg in 1ml
VANCOMYCIN 500mg (Vancocin, Lilly)	0.3ml/500mg	9.7ml water	10ml	50mg in 1ml
Endocrine system				
CALCITONIN 160 units (Calcitare, RPR)	Negligible	1ml diluent	1ml	160 units in 1ml
GLUCAGON 1 unit (Lilly)	0.04ml	0.96ml diluent	1ml	1 unit in 1ml
HYDROCORTISONE SODIUM SUCCINATE 100mg (Solu-Cortef, Upjohn)	0.05ml/100mg	1.95ml water	2ml	50mg in 1ml
LIOTHYRONINE 20μg (Triiodothyronine, Evans)	Zero	1ml water	1ml	20μg in 1ml
METHYLPREDNISOLONE 40mg (Solu-Medrone, Upjohn)	Zero	1ml diluent	1ml	40mg in 1ml
Obstetrics and gynaecology				
INDOMETHACIN 1mg (Indocid PDA, Morson)	Zero	2ml water	2ml	500μg in 1ml
Malignant disease and immunosuppression				
ACLARUBICIN 20mg (Aclacin, Lundbeck)	Zero	10ml water	10ml	2mg in 1ml
ACTINOMYCIN D 500μg (Cosmegen Lyovac, MSD)	Allowed for	1.1ml water		500μg in 1ml
AZATHIOPRINE 50mg (Imuran, Wellcome)	0.05ml/50mg	4.95ml water	5ml	10mg in 1ml
BLEOMYCIN 15 units (Lundbeck)	Weight varies as preparation has been purified. Ampoules contain 7 to 8mg of powder			
CARMUSTINE 100mg (BiCNU, Bristol Myers)	Negligible	3ml diluent then 27ml water	30ml	100mg in 30ml
CORYNEBACTERIUM PARVUM 7mg (Coparavax. Wellcome)	Negligible	1ml sodium chloride 0.9%	1ml	7mg in 1ml

TABLE 10.3 (contd)

Drug	Displacement volume	Reconstitute with	Final volume	Dosage guide
CRISTANTASPASE 10,000 units (Erwinase, Porton)	Zero	1ml water	1ml	10,000 units in 1ml
CYCLOPHOSPHAMIDE 100mg (Farmitalia)	0.1ml/100mg	4.9ml water	5ml	20mg in 1ml
CYTARABINE 100mg (Cytosar, Upjohn)	0.06ml/100mg	4.94ml water	5ml	20mg in 1ml
DACARBAZINE 100mg (DTIC Dome, Bayer)	0.1ml/100mg	9.9ml water	10ml	10mg in 1ml
DOXORUBICIN 10mg (Doxorubicin RD, Farmitalia)	0.03ml/10mg	4.97ml water	5ml	2mg in 1ml
EPIRUBICIN 10mg (Pharmorubicin RD, Farmitalia)	0.03ml/10mg	4.97ml water	5ml	2mg in 1ml
IDARUBICIN 5mg (Zavedos, Farmitalia)	Negligible	5ml water	5ml	1mg in 1ml

IFOSFAMIDE 500mg
(Mitoxana, ASTA)

$$\text{Final volume of solution} = \frac{(\text{Conc. Ifosfamide (\%)} \times \text{ml water added} \times 0.7)}{100} + \text{ml water added}$$

e.g. Add 6.25ml water to 500mg vial to give 8% solution then
$$\text{final volume} = \frac{(8 \times 6.25 \times 0.7)}{100} + 6.25$$
$$= 6.6\text{ml (100mg in 1.32ml)}$$

Drug	Displacement volume	Reconstitute with	Final volume	Dosage guide
INTERFERON 3 megaunits (Intron A, Schering Plough)	Zero	1ml water	1ml	3 megaunits in 1ml
INTERFERON 3 megaunits (Roteron A, Roche)	0.1ml	0.9ml water	1ml	3 megaunits in 1ml
MELPHALAN 100mg (Alkeran, Wellcome)	Negligible	1.8ml Wellcome Acid-Alcohol solvent followed by 9ml Wellcome diluent		100mg in 10.8ml
MITOMYCIN 2mg (Mitomycin C Kyowa, Martindale)	Negligible	5ml water	5ml	400μg in 1ml
MUSTINE 10mg (Boots)	Negligible	10ml water	10ml	1mg in 1ml
PLICAMYCIN 2.5mg (Mithracin, Pfizer)	0.1ml/2.5mg	4.9ml water	5ml	500μg in 1ml

TABLE 10.3 (contd)

Drug	Displacement volume	Reconstitute with	Final volume	Dosage guide
POLYESTRADIOL PHOSPHATE 40mg (Estradurin, Kabi Pharmacia)	0.05 to 0.25ml	2ml water	2.05 to 2.25ml	
THIOTEPA 15mg (Lederle)	0.1ml	1.4ml water	1.5ml	10mg in 1ml
TREOSULPHAN 250mg (Medac)	2.5ml/5g	97.5ml water	100ml	2.5mg in 1ml
VINBLASTINE 10mg (Velbe, Lilly)	Negligible	10ml diluent	10ml	1mg in 1ml
VINDESINE 5mg (Eldisine, Lilly)	Negligible	5ml diluent	5ml	1mg in 1ml
Nutrition and blood DESFERRIOXAMINE 500mg (Desferal, Ciba)	0.4ml/500mg	4.6ml water	5ml	100mg in 1ml
ERYTHROPOIETIN 2,000 units (Recormon, Boehringer Mannheim)	Zero	2ml water	2ml	1,000 units in 1ml
SOLIVITO N (Kabi Pharmacia)	0.3ml	9.7ml water	10ml	
Musculoskeletal and joint diseases HYALURONIDASE 1,500 units (Hyalase, CP)	Zero	1ml water	1ml	1,500 units in 1ml
Anaesthesia METHOHEXITONE 100mg (Brietal Sodium, Lilly)	0.07ml/100mg	9.93ml water	10ml	For a 1% solution
THIOPENTONE 2.5g (Intraval, RPR)	1.5ml/2.5g	98.5ml water	100ml	For a 2.5% solution

Source: Mulholland, P., *Pharmaceutical Journal*, 1993, **251**, 14–15.

ADMINISTRATION OF DRUGS

Oral administration

As stated before, it is not always possible to give tablets or capsules: either the dose required does not exist, or the child cannot swallow tablets or capsules.

Therefore an oral liquid preparation is necessary, either a ready-made preparation, or one made specially by the pharmacy.

TABLE 10.4 Oral syringe volume

Volume	Graduations
0.5 ml	0.01 ml
1.0 ml	0.01 ml or 0.1 ml
2.5 ml	0.25 ml
5.0 ml	0.5 ml
10.0 ml	0.5 ml
20.0 ml	1.0 ml

As you have seen with the examples, not all the doses are convenient 5 ml doses. In these cases an oral syringe is used. There are many oral syringes available, but the are usually available in the volumes shown in Table 10.4.

You should choose the oral syringe most appropriate to the dose you are measuring.

As with syringes for parenteral use, there is a residual volume of liquid left in the nozzle of the syringe. This small volume (0.03 ml) is already taken into account by the manufacturer when calibrating the syringe. Therefore you shouldn't try and administer this small volume: this is known as 'dead space' or 'dead volume'.

A part of their design is that it should not be possible to attach a needle to the nozzle of the oral syringe. This prevents the accidental intravenous administration of an oral preparation.

Intravenous administration (infusions)

It is now commonplace to use infusion pumps when giving infusions as opposed to using a paediatric or microdrop giving set on its own. Using an infusion pump is considered to be more accurate and safer, although using a paediatric giving set on its own still occurs.

With an infusion pump, a 20 drops/ml giving set is usually used, but sometimes a 60 drops/ml microdrop giving set is used.

Infusion rate calculations are quite simple with infusion pumps: rates are usually given in ml/hour, so there isn't any calculation to do.

Make sure that paediatric
doses are checked carefully

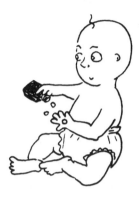

The only time when a calculation might be necessary is to convert dosages to ml/hour (see Section 9 on Intravenous therapy: infusion rate calculations for explanation and examples).

USEFUL REFERENCE BOOKS

1. *Alder Hey Book of Children's Doses*, 6th Edition, Pharmacy Department, Alder Hey Children's Hospital, Liverpool, 1994
2. *A Paediatric Vade-Mecum*, 12th Edition (edited by J. Insley), Edward Arnold, London, 1990
3. *The Paediatric Prescriber*, 5th Edition, Catzel and Oliver, Blackwell Scientific Publications, Oxford, 1981
4. *A Neonatal Pharmacopoeia*, 1993 Edition, Royal Victoria Infirmary, Newcastle upon Tyne, 1993
5. *A Neonatal Vade-Mecum*, 2nd Edition (edited by Fleming, Spiedel, Marlow and Dunn), Edward Arnold, London, 1991
6. *Paediatric Formulary*, 3rd Edition, Pharmacy Department, Guy's Hospital, Lewisham and North Southwark Health Authority, London, 1994

7. *British National Formulary*, Number 29, March 1995, British Medical Association and Royal Pharmaceutical Society of Great Britain, 1995

The latest, up to date, editions should be consulted.

This list is not exhaustive, and there is probably a local in-house reference produced by your hospital. Check your pharmacy department for details.

PROBLEMS

Work out the following dosages, not forgetting to take into account displacement values if necessary.

H.1 Benzylpenicillin at a dose of 25 mg/kg four times a day to a 9-month-old baby weighing 10 kg. How much do you need to draw up for each dose, assuming that each 600 mg vial is to be reconstituted to 2 ml? (N.B. Displacement volume)

H.2 Trimethoprim at a dose of 4 mg/kg twice a day to a 9-year-old child weighing 31.7 kg. Trimethoprim suspension comes as a 50 mg in 5 ml suspension. How much do you need to give for each dose?

H.3 You have to give a dose of salbutamol to a 3-year-old child. The dose on the drug chart is 6 mg, four times a day. However, you think that the dose is rather high and you want to check it. What do you think the dose should be?

(Weight = 15 kg. Dose, from a paediatric reference book = 400 mcg/kg/day in four divided doses)

H.4 Cimetidine syrup is prescribed for a child at a dose of 25 mg/kg/day in four divided doses. How much do you need to give for each doses?

(Weight = 6.4 kg. Cimetidine = 200 mg in 5 ml)

H.5 You need to give cefotaxime I.V. to a 5-year-old child weighing 18 kg at a dose of 150 mg/kg/day in four divided doses. You have a 1 g cefotaxime vial. How much do you need to draw up for each dose? (N.B. Displacement volume)

H.6 You need to give nitrofurantoin suspension at a dose of 3 mg/kg/day in four divided doses to a 12-year-old child weighing 39 kg. You have a 25 mg in 5 ml suspension. How much do you need to give for each dose?

H.7 Using nomograms or tables (see Appendix 1), find out the body surface area for a child weighing 18 kg and with a height of 108 cm.

H.8 Using nomograms or tables (see Appendix 1), find out the body surface area for a child weighing 37 kg and with a height of 148 cm.

H.9 You need to give flucloxacillin I.V. to an 8-year-old child weighing 19.6 kg. The dose is 12.5 mg/kg four times a day. You have a 500 mg vial that needs to be reconstituted to 10 ml with water for injection. How much do you need to draw up? (N.B. Displacement volume)

H.10 You need to give acyclovir to a 12-year-old child with a body surface area of $1.25 \, \text{m}^2$ at a dose of $250 \, \text{mg/m}^2$ every 8 hours. Acyclovir comes as a 250 mg vial and should be given as an infusion over 1 hour at a concentration not more than 5 mg/ml. You need initially to reconstitute each vial with 10 ml water for injection. How much do you need to draw up for each dose and in what volume would you give the infusion? (N.B. Displacement volume)

ANSWERS TO PROBLEMS

H.1 First work out the total dose required:

Dose = 25 mg/kg, Weight = 10 kg

Therefore the total dose equals

$25 \times 10 = 250 \, \text{mg}$

Next, look up the displacement volume for benzylpenicillin. From Table 10.3:

Displacement volume = 0.4 ml/600 mg vial

Work out how much water for injection you need to add to make a final volume of 2 ml, i.e.

$$2\,ml - 0.4\,ml = 1.6\,ml$$

Therefore you need to add 1.6 ml water for injection to each vial to give a final concentration of 600 mg in 2 ml. The next step is to calculate the volume for 250 mg:

600 mg in 2 ml

$$250\,mg = \frac{2}{600} \times 250 = 0.83\,ml$$

Answer: You need to draw up a dose of 250 mg (0.83 ml).

H.2 Dose required = 31.7 × 4 = 127 mg. You have 50 mg in 5 ml. Therefore:

$$127\,mg = \frac{5}{50} \times 127 = 12.7\,ml = 13\,ml\ ('rounding\ up')$$

Answer: You need to give 13 ml of trimethoprim 50 mg in 5 ml.

H.3 Total daily dose = 400 mg/kg/day, weight = 15 kg. Thus *total daily dose* for the child = 400 × 15 = 6,000 mcg = 6 mg. If salbutamol is to be given four times a day (as on the drug chart), then the amount for each dose equals:

$$\frac{6}{4} = 1.5\,mg$$

Therefore the dose should be 1.5 mg four times a day and *not* 6 mg as on the drug chart.

This is a common error made by doctors when calculating doses. The *total daily dose* has been mis-read as each single dose, and consequently the patient will receive too much drug.

CARE MUST BE TAKEN WHEN READING DOSES

H.4 Total daily dose $25 \times 6.4 = 160$ mg. Therefore each dose equals:

$$\frac{160}{4} = 40 \text{ mg (to be given in 4 divided doses)}$$

Cimetidine syrup = 200 mg in 5 ml. Therefore:

$$40 \text{ mg} = \frac{5}{200} \times 40 = 1 \text{ ml}$$

Answer: You need to give 1 ml of cimetidine syrup 200 mg in 5 ml.

H.5 Total daily dose = $18 \times 150 = 2{,}700$ mg. Therefore each dose equals:

$$\frac{2{,}700}{4} = 675 \text{ mg}$$

Displacement volume = 500 mg/0.2 ml, therefore 1 g = 0.4 ml. Add 3.6 ml to a 1 g vial to give 1 g in 4 ml. Thus:

$$675 \text{ mg in } \frac{4}{1{,}000} \times 675 = 2.7 \text{ ml}$$

Answer: You need to draw up 2.7 ml (675 mg).

H.6 Total daily dose = $3 \times 39 = 117$ mg. Therefore each dose equals:

$$\frac{117}{4} = 29.25 \text{ mg} = 30 \text{ mg ('rounding up' for easy calculation)}$$

Sometimes it is necessary to 'adjust' the dose like this for ease of calculation and administration, as long as the 'adjustment' does not make a large difference in the dose.

Suspension = 25 mg in 5 ml. Therefore 30 mg in 6 ml.

Answer: You need to give 6 ml of nitrofurantoin suspension 25 mg in 5 ml.

H.7 0.73 m^2 (using the nomogram)
0.73 m^2 (using the table – 17.5 kg, 110 cm)

H.8 1.25 m^2 (using the nomogram)
1.27 m^2 (using the table – 37.5 kg, 150 cm)

H.9 Dose = 12.5 × 19.6 = 245 mg. Displacement
value = 0.2 ml for 250 mg. Thus for 500 mg = 0.4 ml.
Therefore add 9.6 ml to each vial to give 500 mg in 10 ml.
Thus:

$$245\,\text{mg} = \frac{10}{500} \times 245 = 4.9\,\text{ml}$$

Answer: You need to draw up 4.9 ml.

H.10 Dose = 250 × 1.25 = 312.5 mg. Therefore you need to use
2 vials. The displacement value for acyclovir is negligible,
so add 10 ml water for injection to each vial to give:

250 mg in 10 ml

Volume required for each dose:

$$\frac{10}{250} \times 312.5 = 12.5\,\text{ml}$$

You need to draw up 12.5 ml. The concentration should not
be more than 5 mg/ml. The dose you want is 312.5 mg.
Therefore to find the maximum volume required, divide the
dose by the concentration, i.e.

$$\frac{312.5}{5} = 62.5\,\text{ml}$$

Maximum volume = 62.5 ml. Thus use a 100 ml infusion
bag.

11 Revision test

The purpose of this revision section is to test your ability at drug calculations after you have finished the book.

You should get most, if not all, of the questions right. If you get the wrong answers for any particular section, then you should go back and re-do that section as it indicates that you have not fully understood that type of calculation.

QUESTIONS

Section 2: Basics

The aim of this section is to test your ability on basic principles such as fractions, decimals, powers and using calculators before you start any drug calculations.

Fractions
Solve the following, leaving your answer as a fraction:

1. $\dfrac{5}{16} \times \dfrac{4}{7}$

2. $\dfrac{3}{8} \div \dfrac{6}{7}$

Convert to a decimal:

3. $\dfrac{4}{7}$

Decimals
Solve the following:

    4. 2.15×0.64

    5. $4.2 \div 0.125$

    6. 2.6×100

    7. $45.67 \div 100$

Convert the following to a fraction:

    8. 0.4

Powers
Convert the following to a proper number:

    9. 2.3×10^2

Convert the following number to a power of 10:

    10. 800,000

Section 3: Units and equivalences

This section is designed to re-test your knowledge on units, and
how to convert from one unit to another.

Units of weight

1. 0.125 milligrams	_____	micrograms
2. 0.5 grams	_____	milligrams
3. 0.25 micrograms	_____	nanograms
4. 0.75 kilograms	_____	grams

Units of volume

5. 0.45 litres	_____	millilitres

Units of amount of substance

6. 0.15 moles	_____	millimoles

Section 4: Dosage calculations

Drug dosage

Sometimes the dose is given on a body weight basis or in terms of body surface area. The following tests your ability at calculating doses:

1. Dose = 7.5 mg/kg   Weight = 78 kg
   Dose required = _____ mg

2. Dose = 0.5 mg/kg   Weight = 64 kg
   Dose required = _____ mg

3. Dose = 4 mcg/kg/min   Weight = 56 kg
   Dose required = _____ mcg/min

4. Dose = 4.5 mg/m^2 Surface area = 1.94 m^2
   Dose required = _____ mg

Calculating dosages

Calculate how much you need for the following dosages:

5. You have haloperidol injection 5 mg in 1 ml; amount required = 6 mg.
6. You have atropine injection 600 mcg/1 ml; amount required = 0.1 mg.
7. You have diazepam suspension 2 mg in 5 ml; amount required = 5 mg.
8. You have codeine phosphate syrup 25 mg in 5 ml; amount required = 30 mg.
9. You have potassium chloride injection 1 g in 5 ml ampoules; amount required = 200 mg.
10. You have co-trimoxazole injection 480 mg in 5 ml; amount required = 2,040 mg. What volume and how many ampoules do you need?
11. You have potassium chloride injection 1 g in 5 ml (13.5 mmol in 5 ml); amount required = 10 mmol.
12. You have heparin 1,000 units in 1 ml; amount required = 800 units.

Section 5: Percent and percentages

Convert the following fractions into percentages:

1. $\dfrac{7}{20}$ _____ %

2. $\dfrac{1}{8}$ _____ %

Convert each of the following percentages to a fraction in its simplest form:

3. 45%
4. 60%

Convert the following decimals into percentages:

5. 0.23 _____ %
6. 4.075 _____ %

Convert the following percentages to a decimal:

7. 30%
8. 57.5%

Drug calculations involving percentages

9. How much is 28% of 250 g
10. What percentage is 160 g of 400 g?

Section 6: Drug strengths or concentrations

This section is designed to see if you understood the various ways in which drug strengths can be expressed.

Percentage concentration

1. How much glucose (in grams) is there in a 500 ml infusion of glucose 10%
2. You need to add 1.5 g of potassium chloride to a litre of sodium chloride 0.9% infusion. You have 10 ml ampoules of 20% potassium chloride. What volume of potassium chloride do you need to draw up?

mg/ml concentrations

3. What is the concentration (in mg/ml) of a 30% sodium chloride ampoule?
4. You need to give a 300 mg dose of rifampicin to a patient. You have a bottle of rifampicin suspension at concentration of 20 mg/ml. How much do you need to give for your dose?

'1 in ...' concentrations or ratio strengths

5. You have a 1 ml ampoule of adrenaline 1 in 1,000. How much adrenaline (in milligrams) does the ampoule contain?

Drugs expressed in units

6. You need to give an infusion of heparin containing 32,000 units over 24 hours. You have ampoules of heparin containing 25,000 units/ml and 5,000 units/ml. How much of each ampoule do you need to draw up?

Section 7: Preparation of solutions (dilutions)

This section is designed to see if you learnt how to do simple dilutions when making solutions of varying strengths and how to prepare solutions for soaks.

Preparation of simple solutions

1. You are asked to prepare 250 ml of a 40% solution. How much of your stock solution do you need which diluted to 250 ml will give a 40% solution?
2. You are asked to prepare 200 ml of a 60% solution from an 80% stock solution. How much of your stock solution do you need which diluted to 200 ml will give a 60% solution?

Preparation of soaks

3. You are asked to prepare 1,000 ml of a 1 in 8,000 solution of potassium permanganate for a soak. You have

a solution of potassium permanganate 1%. How much of your stock solution do you need to dilute to make 1,000 ml of your soak?

4. You are asked to prepare 250 ml of a 1 in 10,000 solution of potassium permanganate for a soak. You have a solution of potassium permanganate 1 in 2,000. How much of your stock solution do you need to dilute to make 250 ml of your soak?

Section 8: Moles and millimoles

This section is designed to see if you understood the concept of millimoles.

Note that the molecular weight of sodium bicarbonate is 84, and the molecular weight of sodium chloride is 58.5

1. Approximately how many millimoles of sodium are there in a 200 ml infusion of sodium bicarbonate 8.4%?
2. Approximately how many mmol per litre of sodium are there in an infusion containing 4.5 g of sodium chloride per litre?

Section 9: Infusion rate calculations

This section tests your knowledge of various infusion rate calculations. It is designed to see if you know the different drop factors for different giving sets and fluids, as well as being able to convert volumes to drops and vice versa.

Calculation of drip rates

1. What is the rate required to give 1 litre of glucose 5% infusion over 6 hours using a standard giving set?
2. What is the rate required to give 1 litre of sodium chloride 0.9% infusion over 8 hours using a standard giving set?
3. What is the rate required to give 1 unit of blood (500 ml) over 6 hours using a standard giving set?

Conversion of infusion rates (ml/hour) to drops/min

4. You are asked to give a 1 litre infusion of sodium chloride 0.9% at a rate of 100 ml/hour using a standard giving set. What is the rate in drops/min?

5. You are asked to give an infusion of 5% glucose at a rate of 2 ml/min using a standard giving set. What is the rate in drops/min?

6. You are asked to give an infusion of isosorbide dinitrate 50 mg in 500 ml glucose 5% at a rate of 4 mg/hour. What is the rate in drops/min?

Conversion of dosages to drops/min and ml/hour

7. You are asked to give 500 ml of doxapram 0.2% infusion at a rate of 1.5 mg/min using a standard giving set. What is the rate in drops/min? What is the rate in ml/hour?

8. You have an infusion of dopamine 800 mg in 500 ml. The dose required is 5 mcg/kg/min and the patient weighs 68 kg. What is the rate in drops/min (using a microdrop giving set)? What is the rate in ml/hour?

9. You have an infusion of nitroprusside 50 mg in 500 ml. The dose required is 4 mcg/kg/min and the patient weighs 72 kg. What is the rate in drops/min (using a standard giving set)? What is the rate in ml/hour?

10. You are asked to give 500 ml of lignocaine 0.2% infusion at a rate of 3 mg/min using a standard giving set. What is the rate in drops/min? What is the rate in ml/hour?

11. You have an infusion of dobutamine 250 mg in 250 ml. The dose required is 6 mcg/kg/min and the patient weighs 77 kg. What is the rate in drops/min (using a microdrop giving set)? What is the rate in ml/hour?

Conversion of ml/hour to mcg/kg/min or mg/min

12. An infusion pump containing 50 mg of sodium nitroprusside in 50 ml, is running at a rate of

18 ml/hour. The dose wanted is 4 mcg/kg/min and the patient's weight is 75 kg. Is the pump rate correct?

13. An infusion pump containing 50 mg of glyceryl trinitrate in 100 ml, is running at a rate of 8 ml/hour. The dose wanted is 4 mg/hour. Is the pump rate correct?

Calculation of length of time of infusions

14. You have a 500 ml infusion at a rate of 21 drops/min using a standard giving set. Approximately how long will the infusion run?

15. A patient has a high serum calcium level. You have an infusion of disodium pamidronate 15 mg in 250 ml. The infusion should not take less than an hour. The rate at which the infusion is running, using a standard giving set, equals 42 drops/min. How long will the infusion take?

Section 10: Paediatric dosage calculations

1. You need to give salbutamol to a 5-year-old child weighing 18 kg at a dose of 100 mcg/kg four times a day. Salbutamol comes as a 2 mg in 5 ml syrup. How much do you need for each dose?

2. You need to give benzylpenicillin at a dose of 25 mg/kg four times a day to a year old baby weighing 11 kg. How much do you need to draw up for each dose assuming each 600 mg vial is to be reconstituted to 2 ml?

ANSWERS

Section 2: Basics

Fractions

1. $\dfrac{5}{28}$

2. $\dfrac{7}{16}$

3. 0.57

Decimals

4. 1.376
5. 33.6
6. 260
7. 0.4567
8. $\frac{2}{5}$

Powers

9. 230
10. 8×10^5

Section 3: Units and equivalences

Units of weight

1. 125 micrograms
2. 500 milligrams
3. 250 nanograms
4. 750 grams

Units of volume

5. 450 millilitres

Units of amount of substance

6. 150 millimoles

Section 4: Dosage calculations

Drug dosage

1. 585 mg
2. 32 mg
3. 224 mcg/min
4. 8.73 mg

Calculating dosages

   5. 1.2 ml
   6. 0.17 ml
   7. 12.5 ml
   8. 6 ml
   9. 1 ml
  10. 21.25 ml; 5 ampoules
  11. 3.7 ml
  12. 0.8 ml

Section 5: Percent and percentages

   1. 35%
   2. 12.5%
   3. $\dfrac{9}{20}$
   4. $\dfrac{3}{5}$
   5. 23%
   6. 407.5%
   7. 0.3
   8. 0.575
   9. 70 g
  10. 40%

Section 6: Drug strengths or concentrations

Percentage concentration

   1. 50 g
   2. 7.5 ml

mg/ml concentrations

   3. 300 mg/ml
   4. 15 ml

'1 in ...' concentrations or ratio strengths

   5. 1 mg

Drugs expressed in units

    6. 1 × 25,000 units/ml ampoule *plus*
       1 × 5,000 units/ml ampoule *plus*
       0.4 ml of a 5,000 units/ml ampoule

Section 7: Preparation of solutions (dilutions)

Preparation of simple solutions

    1. 100 ml
    2. 150 ml

Preparation of soaks

    3. 12.5 ml
    4. 50 ml

Section 8: Moles and millimoles

    1. 200 mmol
    2. 77 mmol

Section 9: Infusion rate calculations

Calculation of drip rates

    1. 55.5 drops/min (56 drops/min)
    2. 41.7 drops/min (42 drops/min)
    3. 20.8 drops/min (21 drops/min)

Conversion of infusion rates (ml/hour) to drops/min

    4. 33.3 drops/min (33 drops/min)
    5. 40 drops/min
    6. 13.3 drops/min (13 drops/min)

Conversion of dosages to drops/min and ml/hour

    7. Standard giving set: 15 drops/min; 45 ml/hour
    8. Micro-drop giving set: 12.75 drops/min (13 drops/min);
       12.75 ml/hour

9. Standard giving set: 57.6 drops/min (58 drops/min); 172.8 ml/hour
10. Standard giving set: 30 drops/min; 90 ml/hour
11. Microdrop giving set: 27.72 drops/min (28 drops/min); 27.72 ml/hour

Conversion of ml/hour to mcg/kg/min or mg/min

12. Dose = 18 ml/hour, so the pump rate is correct.
13. Dose = 8 ml/hour, so the pump rate is correct.

Calculation of length of time of infusions

14. 476 min = 7 hours 56 min (approx. 8 hours)
15. 2 hours

Section 10: Paediatric dosage calculations

1. 1.8 mg = 4.5 ml
2. 0.92 ml

APPENDIX 1
Body surface area estimates
••

NOMOGRAMS

This is the usual method for calculating body surface area.

Figures A1.1 and A1.2 are nomograms for estimating body surface area in children and adults.

Once the height and weight are known, a straight line edge (e.g. a ruler) is placed from the patient's height in the left column to his/her weight in the right column and the intersect on the body surface area column indicates the body surface area (see Figure A1.3).

For example, you want to know the body surface area of a child weighing 16.4 kg whose height is 100.5 cm.

Align the left-hand side of the ruler against the 100 cm mark on the left-hand column (nearest point to 100.5 cm). Next, align the right-hand side of the ruler to 16.5 kg on the right column (nearest point to 16.4 kg). Now read off where the ruler intersects the body surface area column. In this case it is 0.66 m².

TABLES

Once again, height and weight are measured and the corresponding body surface area is read from Table A1.1 (feet and pounds) or Table A1.2 (centimetres and kilograms). *In both cases the surface area is shown in square metres.*

Using our original example (weight = 16.4 kg, height = 100.5 cm), go down the left-hand (Weight) column of Table A1.2 until you reach 17.5 kg (nearest to 16.4 kg); then go along the top (Height) line until you reach 100 cm (nearest to 100.5 cm). Then read off the corresponding body surface area. In this case it equals 0.68 m². This is shown in Table A1.3.

Both methods give a reasonable estimate of body surface area.

TABLE A1.3

Height (cm)	90	95	100	105	110
Weight (kg)					
10	0.50	0.52	0.54	0.56	
12.5	0.55	0.57	0.59	0.61	0.64
15	0.59	0.62	0.64	0.66	0.69
17.5	0.63	0.66	(0.68)	0.71	0.73
20	0.67	0.70	0.72	0.75	0.78

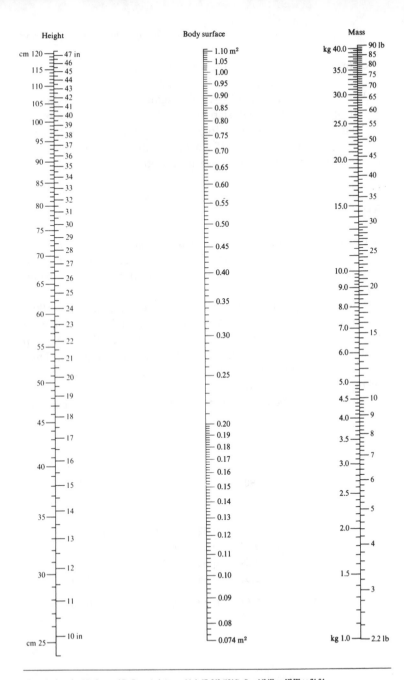

Height	Body surface	Mass

Height
cm 120 — 47 in
46
115 — 45
44
110 — 43
42
105 — 41
40
100 — 39
38
95 — 37
36
90 — 35
34
85 — 33
32
80 — 31
30
75 — 29
28
70 — 27
26
65 — 25
24
60 — 23
22
55 — 21
20
50 — 19
18
45 — 17
16
40 — 15
14
35 — 13
12
30 — 11
cm 25 — 10 in

Body surface
1.10 m²
1.05
1.00
0.95
0.90
0.85
0.80
0.75
0.70
0.65
0.60
0.55
0.50
0.45
0.40
0.35
0.30
0.25
0.20
0.19
0.18
0.17
0.16
0.15
0.14
0.13
0.12
0.11
0.10
0.09
0.08
0.074 m²

Mass
kg 40.0 — 90 lb
85
35.0 — 80
75
30.0 — 70
65
25.0 — 60
55
50
20.0 — 45
40
15.0 — 35
30
25
10.0
9.0 — 20
8.0
7.0 — 15
6.0
5.0
4.5 — 10
4.0 — 9
3.5 — 8
3.0 — 7
6
2.5 — 5
2.0 — 4
1.5 — 3
kg 1.0 — 2.2 lb

¹ From the formula of Du Bois and Du Bois, *Arch. intern. Med.*, **17**, 863 (1916): $S = M^{0.425} \times H^{0.725} \times 71.84$, or $\log S = \log M \times 0.425 + \log H \times 0.725 + 1.8564$ (S: body surface in cm², M: mass in kg, H: height in cm).

FIGURE A1.1 Nomogram for estimating body surface area in children (From: *Scientific Tables*, K. Diem and C. Lentner, 7th edn, 1970, Basle, J.R. Geigy)

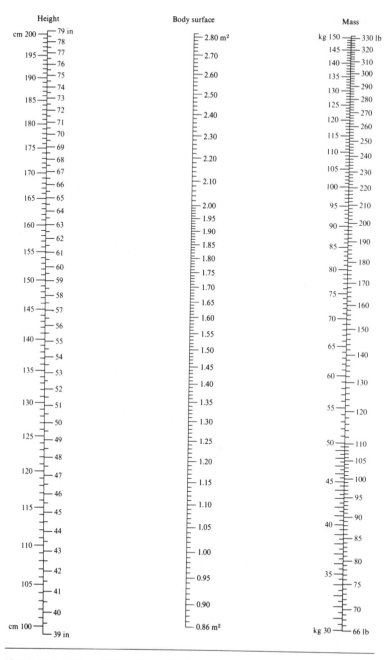

† From the formula of Du Bois and Du Bois, *Arch. intern. Med.*, **17**, 863 (1916): $S = M^{0.425} \times H^{0.725} \times 71.84$, or $\log S = \log M \times 0.425 + \log H \times 0.725 + 1.8564$ (S: body surface in cm², M: mass in kg, H: height in cm).

FIGURE A1.2 Nomogram for estimating body surface area in adults (From: *Scientific Tables*, K. Diem and C. Lentner, 7th edn, 1970, Basle, J.R. Geigy)

TABLE A1.1 Body surface area (square metres) for a given height (feet and inches) and weight (pounds)

Weight (lb)	3'0"	3'2"	3'4"	3'6"	3'8"	3'10"	4'0"	4'2"	4'4"	4'6"	4'8"	4'10"	5'0"	5'2"	5'4"	5'6"	5'8"	5'10"	6'0"	6'2"	6'4"	6'6"
14	0.42																					
21	0.50	0.51																				
28	0.56	0.58	0.60	0.63																		
35	0.62	0.64	0.66	0.69	0.71	0.73																
42	0.66	0.69	0.72	0.74	0.77	0.79	0.82	0.84														
49		0.74	0.77	0.79	0.82	0.85	0.87	0.90	0.93													
56		0.78	0.81	0.84	0.87	0.90	0.92	0.95	0.98	1.01												
63				0.88	0.91	0.94	0.97	1.00	1.03	1.06	1.09											
70					0.95	0.98	1.02	1.05	1.08	1.11	1.14											
77					0.99	1.03	1.06	1.09	1.12	1.15	1.18	1.21	1.25	1.28								
84						1.06	1.10	1.13	1.16	1.20	1.23	1.26	1.29	1.32	1.35							
91							1.14	1.17	1.20	1.24	1.27	1.30	1.34	1.37	1.40	1.43	1.46					
98								1.21	1.24	1.28	1.31	1.35	1.38	1.41	1.45	1.48	1.51	1.54				
105								1.24	1.28	1.32	1.35	1.39	1.42	1.45	1.49	1.52	1.55	1.59	1.62			
112											1.39	1.42	1.46	1.50	1.53	1.56	1.60	1.63	1.67	1.70		
119											1.42	1.46	1.50	1.53	1.57	1.60	1.64	1.67	1.71	1.74	1.78	

126	1.46	1.50	1.53	1.57	1.61	1.64	1.68	1.72	1.75	1.79	1.82	1.86
133		1.53	1.57	1.61	1.65	1.68	1.72	1.76	1.79	1.83	1.86	1.90
140		1.57	1.60	1.64	1.68	1.72	1.76	1.79	1.83	1.87	1.90	1.94
147			1.64	1.68	1.72	1.76	1.79	1.83	1.87	1.91	1.94	1.98
154				1.71	1.75	1.79	1.83	1.87	1.91	1.95	1.98	2.02
161				1.74	1.78	1.82	1.86	1.90	1.94	1.98	2.02	2.06
168					1.82	1.86	1.90	1.94	1.98	2.02	2.06	2.10
175					1.85	1.89	1.93	1.97	2.01	2.05	2.09	2.13
182					1.92	1.96	2.01	2.05	2.09	2.13	2.17	
189					1.95	2.00	2.04	2.08	2.12	2.16	2.21	
196						2.03	2.07	2.11	2.16	2.20	2.24	
203						2.06	2.10	2.14	2.19	2.23	2.27	
210							2.13	2.18	2.22	2.26	2.31	
217							2.16	2.21	2.25	2.29	2.34	
224								2.24	2.28	2.33	2.37	
231									2.31	2.36	2.40	
238										2.39	2.43	

Source: *Martindale: The Extra Pharmacopoeia*, ed. A. Wade and J.E.F. Reynolds, 27th edn, 1977, London, Pharmaceutical Press

TABLE A1.2 Body surface area (square metres) for a given height (centimetres) and weight (kilograms)

Height (cm)	90	95	100	105	110	115	120	125	130	135	140	145	150	155	160	165	170	175	180	185	190	195
Weight (kg)																						
10	0.50	0.52	0.54	0.56																		
12.5	0.55	0.57	0.59	0.61	0.64																	
15	0.59	0.62	0.64	0.66	0.69	0.71	0.73															
17.5	0.63	0.66	0.68	0.71	0.73	0.76	0.78	0.80														
20	0.67	0.70	0.72	0.75	0.78	0.80	0.83	0.85	0.88	0.90												
22.5			0.76	0.79	0.82	0.84	0.87	0.89	0.92	0.95	0.97	1.00										
25				0.82	0.85	0.88	0.91	0.94	0.96	0.99	1.02	1.04	1.07									
27.5				0.86	0.89	0.92	0.95	0.97	1.00	1.03	1.06	1.08	1.11	1.14	1.16							
30					0.92	0.95	0.98	1.01	1.04	1.07	1.10	1.13	1.15	1.18	1.21	1.24						
32.5					0.95	0.98	1.02	1.05	1.08	1.11	1.14	1.16	1.19	1.22	1.25	1.28	1.31					
35						1.02	1.05	1.08	1.11	1.14	1.17	1.20	1.23	1.26	1.29	1.32	1.35					
37.5							1.08	1.11	1.14	1.17	1.21	1.24	1.27	1.30	1.33	1.36	1.39	1.42				
40								1.14	1.17	1.21	1.24	1.27	1.30	1.33	1.37	1.40	1.43	1.46				
42.5								1.17	1.21	1.24	1.27	1.30	1.34	1.37	1.40	1.43	1.46	1.50	1.53			
45									1.24	1.27	1.30	1.34	1.37	1.40	1.44	1.47	1.50	1.53	1.56			
47.5									1.26	1.30	1.33	1.37	1.40	1.44	1.47	1.50	1.53	1.57	1.60	1.63		
50									1.29	1.33	1.36	1.40	1.43	1.47	1.50	1.54	1.57	1.60	1.64	1.67	1.70	
52.5										1.36	1.39	1.43	1.46	1.50	1.53	1.57	1.60	1.64	1.67	1.70	1.74	1.77
55										1.38	1.42	1.46	1.49	1.53	1.56	1.60	1.63	1.67	1.70	1.74	1.77	1.80
57.5											1.45	1.48	1.52	1.56	1.59	1.63	1.66	1.70	1.74	1.77	1.80	1.84

60	1.47	1.51	1.55	1.59	1.62	1.66	1.70	1.73	1.77	1.80	1.84	1.87
62.5		1.54	1.58	1.61	1.65	1.69	1.72	1.76	1.80	1.83	1.87	1.91
65		1.56	1.60	1.64	1.68	1.72	1.75	1.79	1.83	1.86	1.90	1.94
67.5			1.63	1.67	1.71	1.74	1.78	1.82	1.86	1.90	1.93	1.97
70			1.65	1.69	1.73	1.77	1.81	1.85	1.89	1.92	1.96	2.00
72.5				1.72	1.76	1.80	1.84	1.88	1.91	1.95	1.99	2.03
75				1.74	1.78	1.82	1.86	1.90	1.94	1.98	2.02	2.06
77.5					1.81	1.85	1.89	1.93	1.97	2.01	2.05	2.09
80					1.83	1.87	1.92	1.96	2.00	2.04	2.08	2.12
82.5						1.90	1.94	1.98	2.02	2.06	2.10	2.14
85							1.96	2.01	2.05	2.09	2.13	2.17
87.5							1.99	2.03	2.07	2.12	2.16	2.20
90								2.06	2.10	2.14	2.18	2.22
92.5								2.08	2.12	2.17	2.21	2.25
95									2.15	2.19	2.23	2.28
97.5									2.17	2.22	2.26	2.30
100										2.24	2.28	2.33
102.5										2.26	2.31	2.35
105											2.33	2.38
107.5												2.40

Source: Martindale: The Extra Pharmacopoeia, ed. A. Wade and J.E.F. Reynolds, 27th edn, 1977, London, Pharmaceutical Press

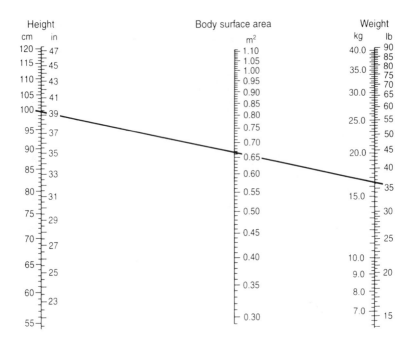

FIGURE A1.3 Nomogram for determination of body surface area from height and weight (From: *Scientific Tables*, K. Diem and C. Lentner, 7th edn, 1970, Basle, J.R. Geigy)

APPENDIX 2

Weight and height conversions

....

WEIGHT CONVERSION TABLES

Sometimes, it may be necessary to convert stones and pounds to kilograms and vice versa. Patients' weights are usually given in stones and have to be converted to kilograms, especially when working out dosages. A lot of dosages are calculated on a 'weight basis', e.g. mg/kg/day. Table A2.1 shows weight conversions.

WORKED EXAMPLE

Convert 14 stones 4 pounds to kilograms (to the nearest kg).

1. Using the conversion table:

14 stones	$= 88.9\,kg$
4 pounds	$= \underline{\ 1.8\,kg}$
	$90.7\,kg$
Answer:	91 kg (to nearest kg)

2. Using the conversion factors: STONES TO KILOGRAMS (multipy by 6.3503)

14 stones $= 14 \times 6.3503 = 88.9042\,kg$

POUNDS TO KILOGRAMS (multiply by 0.4536)

4 pounds $= 4 \times 0.4536$	$=\ 1.8144\,kg$
Add the two together:	$88.9042\,kg$
	$\underline{\ 1.8144\,kg}$
	$90.7186\,kg$
Answer:	91 kg (to nearest kg)

TABLE A2.1

STONES TO KILOGRAMS		POUNDS TO KILOGRAMS	
Stones	Kilograms	Pounds	Kilograms
1	6.4	1	0.5
2	12.7	2	0.9
3	19.1	3	1.4
4	25.4	4	1.8
5	31.8	5	2.3
6	38.1	6	2.7
7	44.5	7	3.2
8	50.8	8	3.6
9	57.2	9	4.1
10	63.5	10	4.5
11	69.9	11	5.0
12	76.2	12	5.4
13	82.6	13	5.9
14	88.9		
15	95.3		
16	101.6		
17	108.0		
18	114.3		
19	120.7		
20	127.0		

Weights in kg correct to 0.1 kg

Conversion factors

Stones to kilograms × 6.3503
Pounds to kilograms × 0.4536

Kilograms to stones × 0.1575
Kilograms to pounds × 2.2046

HEIGHT CONVERSION TABLES

Sometimes, it may be necessary to convert feet and inches to centimetres and vice versa. Patients' heights are usually given in feet and inches and have to be converted to centimetres. Some dosages are calculated on a 'surface area basis', e.g. mg/m^2, particularly cytotoxic drugs. Table A2.2 shows height conversions.

TABLE A2.2

FEET TO CENTIMETRES		INCHES TO CENTIMETRES	
Feet	Centimetres	Inches	Centimetres
1	30.5	1	2.5
2	61.0	2	5.1
3	91.4	3	7.6
4	121.9	4	10.2
5	152.4	5	12.7
6	182.9	6	15.2
7	213.4	7	17.8
8	243.8	8	20.3
		9	22.9
Lengths in cm correct to 0.1 cm		10	25.4
		11	27.9

Conversion factors

Feet to centimetres × 30.48   Centimetres to feet × 0.028
Inches to centimetres × 2.54   Centimetres to inches × 0.3937

WORKED EXAMPLE

Convert 6 feet 2 inches to centimetres (to the nearest cm).

1. Using the conversion table:

6 feet	= 182.9 cm
2 inches	= 5.1 cm
	188.0 cm
Answer:	188 cm (to nearest cm)

2. Using the conversion factors: FEET TO CENTIMETRES (multiply by 30.48)

6 feet = 6 × 30.48   = 182.88 cm

INCHES TO CENTIMETRES (multiply by 2.54)

2 inches = 2 × 2.54   =   5.08 cm
Add the two together: 182.88 cm
                          5.08 cm
                        187.96 cm

Answer: 188 cm (to nearest cm)

Preparation of powders
••

TRITURATION

Sometimes the dose required can be extremely small – too small to be given in the form of tablets or made into syrups or suspensions because they are unstable.

When this occurs, the powder form of the medicine is diluted with an inert substance, such as lactose, and dispensed as individual doses or powders.

This process of dilution is called **trituration**, and several triturations may be required if the dose is very small or if a potent drug is involved; for example, doses in neonates and paediatrics.

There are two methods for preparing powders:

1. Dilution of the drug as a powder
2. Weighing and crushing tablets, then diluting with a suitable diluent.

Method one: Dilution of the medicine as a powder

WORKED EXAMPLE

A child needs thyroxine at a dose of 35 mcg. This is too small to be given in the form of tablets, and a suspension cannot be made. Therefore powders need to be prepared. You need 14 powders.

To allow for wastage, you usually calculate for an extra two powders. Thus in this case, calculate for 16 powders.

Step 1
Calculate the total amount of drug required for 16 powders, i.e. each powder is to contain 35 mcg, therefore for 16 powders you will need:

$16 \times 35 = 560$ mcg (0.56 mg)

It is impossible to weigh 560 mcg, let alone divide into 16 equal amounts. Therefore it is necessary to use a larger weighable amount and then dilute it by trituration.

Step 2
On a normal dispensing balance, it is good dispensing practice never to weigh less than 100 mg (Class B balance). Therefore each final powder must weigh at least 100 mg. Calculate the total amount for the number of powders required (16), i.e.

16×100 mg $= 1,600$ mg

Step 3
Therefore it is necessary to dilute the drug until you have a final powder weighing 100 mg that contains 35 mcg of drug (this may take several dilutions or triturations).
Dilution 1 (1 in 50 dilution):

Thyroxine	100 mg	(minimum weighable amount)
Lactose	4,900 mg	
	5,000 mg	

Each 100 mg of this dilution will contain 2 mg of thyroxine. You have 100 mg thyroxine in 5,000 mg, therefore in 100 mg there are:

$$\frac{100}{5,000} \times 100 = 2 \text{ mg}$$

Step 4
It is necessary to make a further dilution.
Dilution 2 (1 in 20 dilution):

From dilution 1	100 mg	$(= 2 \text{ mg thyroxine})$
Lactose	1,900 mg	
	2,000 mg	

Each 100 mg of this dilution will contain 0.1 mg (100 mcg) of thyroxine. You have 2 mg thyroxine in 2,000 mg, therefore in 100 mg there are:

$$\frac{2}{2,000} \times 100 = 0.1 \text{ mg (100 mcg)}$$

Step 5

You have already calculated that you need a final amount of 560 mcg of thyroxine (from step 1).

You know that 100 mg of powder from dilution 2 contains 100 mcg of thyroxine, thus for 560 mcg you will need 560 mg of powder (from dilution 2).

The total amount required for 16 powders (step 2) is 1,600 mg. Therefore, take 560 mg from dilution 2 and make up to 1,600 mg.

Dilution 3 (dilution according to the dose required):

From dilution 2	560 mg	(= 560 mcg of thyroxine)
Lactose	1,040 mg	(1,600 mg − 560 mg)
	1,600 mg	

Each 100 mg of this final dilution will contain 35 mcg of thyroxine. You have 560 mcg thyroxine in 1,600 mg, therefore in 100 mg there are:

$$\frac{560}{1,600} \times 100 = 35 \text{ mcg}$$

Therefore weigh 14 lots of 100 mg (as required).

Other 'doses' of varying strengths

If the dose required is in terms of 'hundreds of micrograms' ($\times$ 100 mcg) or 'units of milligrams' ($\times$ 1 mg) instead of 'tens of micrograms' ($\times$ 10 mcg), then the same methods are used but different dilutions are made.

1. *'Hundreds of micrograms'* ($\times$ 100 mcg):

   Dilution 1 = 1 in 20 dilution (100 mg diluted to 2,000 mg)
   Dilution 2 = 1 in 5 dilution (100 mg diluted to 500 mg)
   Dilution 3 = dilution according to dose required

2. *'Units of milligrams'* ($\times$ 1 mg):

   Dilution 1 = 1 in 10 dilution (100 mg diluted to 1,000 mg)
   Dilution 2 = dilution according to dose required

WORKED EXAMPLES

1. *'Hundreds of micrograms'* (× 100 mcg)

Dose required = hyoscine 600 mcg, and you need 10 powders.

Dilution 1 (1 in 20 dilution):

Hyoscine	100 mg
Lactose	1,900 mg
	2,000 mg

Each 100 mg of this dilution contains 5 mg of hyoscine. You have 100 mg hyoscine in 2,000 mg, therefore in 100 mg there are:

$$\frac{100}{2,000} \times 100 = 5 \text{ mg}$$

Dilution 2 (1 in 5 dilution):

From dilution 1	200 mg	(= 10 mg of hyoscine)
Lactose	800 mg	
	1,000 mg	

Each 100 mg of this dilution contains 1 mg of hyoscine. You have 10 mg hyoscine in 1,000 mg, therefore in 100 mg there are:

$$\frac{10}{1,000} \times 100 = 1 \text{ mg}$$

Dilution 3 (dilution according to the dose required):

In this example the dose required is hyoscine 600 mcg, making 10 powders. Total dose required = 600 mcg × 10 = 6 mg.

Take 600 mg from dilution 2 (= 6 mg of hyoscine) and dilute to 1,000 mg (10 powders of 100 mg = 1,000 mg):

From dilution 2	600 mg	(= 6 mg of hyoscine)
Lactose	400 mg	(1,000 mg − 600 mg)
	1,000 mg	

Each 100 mg of this dilution contains 0.6 mg (600 mcg) of hyoscine. You have 6 mg hyoscine in 1,000 mg, therefore in 100 mg there are:

$$\frac{6}{1,000} \times 100 = 0.6 \text{ mg } (600 \text{ mcg})$$

2. *'Units of milligrams' ($\times$ 1 mg)*

Dose required = codeine phosphate 1.5 mg, and you need 10 powders.

Dilution 1 (1 in 10 dilution):

Codeine phosphate	100 mg
Lactose	900 mg
	1,000 mg

Each 100 mg of this dilution contains 10 mg of codeine phosphate. You have 100 mg codeine phosphate in 1,000 mg, therefore in 100 mg there are:

$$\frac{100}{1,000} \times 100 = 10 \text{ mg}$$

Dilution 2 (dilution according to the dose required)

In this example the dose required is codeine phosphate 1.5 mg, making 10 powders. Total dose required = 1.5 mg $\times$ 10 = 15 mg.

Take 150 mg from dilution 1 (= 15 mg of codeine phosphate) and dilute to 1,000 mg (10 powders of 100 mg = 1,000 mg):

From dilution 1	150 mg	(= 15 mg of codeine phosphate)
Lactose	850 mg	(1,000 mg − 150 mg)
	1,000 mg	

Each 100 mg of this dilution contains 1.5 mg of codeine phosphate. You have 15 mg codeine phosphate in 1,000 mg, therefore in 100 mg there are:

$$\frac{15}{1,000} \times 100 = 1.5 \text{ mg}$$

Method two: weighing and crushing tablets

The advantage of this method is that the drug is readily available in a tablet form, whereas it may not be available, or readily available, in a powdered form.

WORKED EXAMPLE

We use the same worked example as before: a dose of 35 mcg of thyroxine is needed for a child. You need to prepare 14 powders.

Step 1
You need 14 powders, so once again prepare 2 extra (16 powders) to allow for wastage. First work out the total dose for 16 powders:

$$16 \times 35 = 560 \text{ mcg}$$

Step 2
Thyroxine tablets are available in the following strengths: 25 mcg, 50 mcg and 100 mcg.

Obviously, using the above strengths of thyroxine tablets, it is impossible to get the required dose of 560 mcg. The nearest possible dose is either:

(i) 550 mcg = 5 × 100 mcg + 1 × 50 mcg, or
(ii) 575 mcg = 5 × 100 mcg + 1 × 50 mcg + 1 × 25 mcg

If is not possible to match the calculated dose exactly, then it is better to go slightly higher, rather than slightly lower.

Step 3
Next work out the number of powders for the nearest (new) total, i.e. divide the new total dose by the dose required:

$$\frac{575}{35} = 16.43 \text{ powders}$$

So 575 mcg of thyroxine is sufficient to provide 16.43 powders.

Step 4

Now work out the total amount required for the final number of powders. Each powder is to weigh 100 mg, so 16.43 powders will equal:

$$16.43 \times 100 = 1,643 \text{ mg}$$

Step 5

Weigh the tablets and make up to the final amount required (1,643 mg) with lactose.

Weight of 5×100 mcg + 1×50 mcg +
1×25 mcg
$$= 0.7028 \text{ g}$$
$$= 702.8 \text{ mg}$$
$$= 703 \text{ mg}$$

Tablets	703 mg	(contains 575 mcg of thyroxine)
Lactose	940 mg	(1,643 mg − 703 mg)
	1,643 mg	

Each 100 mg of this final dilution will contain 35 mcg of thyroxine. You have 575 mcg thyroxine in 1,643 mg, therefore in 100 mg there are:

$$\frac{575}{1,643} \times 100 = 35 \text{ mcg}$$

Therefore weigh 14 lots of 100 mg (as required).

Abbreviations used in prescriptions

....

Although directions should preferably be in English without abbreviation, it is recognised that some Latin abbreviations are used.

The following is a list of abbreviations that are commonly used.

N.B. Some of these abbreviations may differ as they depend on local convention.

Abbreviation	Latin derivation	English meaning
a.c.	ante cibum	before food
alt die	alterna die	on alternate days
applic.	applicatio	an application
aurist.	auristillae	ear drops
b.d.	bis die	twice daily
b.i.d.	bis in die	twice a day
c or c̄	cum	with
c.c.	cum cibum	with food
		(also: cubic centimetre)
crem.	cremor	a cream
d	dies	daily
elix.		elixir
gtt. (g.)	guttae	drops
h	hors	hour/at the hour of
h.s.	hora somni	at bedtime
I.M.		intramuscular
INH		inhaler/to be inhaled
inj.	injectio	an injection

Abbreviation	Latin derivation	English meaning
irrig.	*irrigatio*	an irrigation
I.U.		International Units
I.V.		intravenous
m	*mane*	morning
m.d.u.	*more dictus utendus*	to be used/taken as directed
mist.	*mistura*	mixture
mitte		send (number of tablets etc. to be dispensed)
n	*nocte*	night
NEB		nebuliser/to be nebulised/nebules
o	*omni*	every
oculent. (oc.)	*oculentum*	eye ointment
o.d.	*omni die*	every day (daily)
o.m.	*omni mane*	every morning
o.n.	*omni nocte*	every night
p.c.	*post cibum*	after food
p.o.	*per os*	orally
p.r.	*per rectum*	rectally
p.r.n.	*pro re nata*	occasionally/when required
p.v.	*per vagina*	vaginally
q	*quaque*	each/every
q6h		every six hours
q.d.s.	*quater die sumendus*	to be taken four times a day
q.i.d.	*quater in die*	four times a day
R		'recipe' = take
s or $\bar{s}$	*sine*	without
S.C.		subcutaneous
sig.	*signa*	let it be labelled
S.L.		sublingual
s.o.s.	*si opus sit*	if required
stat.	*statum*	at once
supp.	*suppositorium*	a suppository
T.D.D.		total daily dose

Abbreviation	Latin derivation	English meaning
t.d.s.	*ter die sumendus*	to be taken three times a day
t.i.d.	*ter in die*	three times a day
TOP		topically
U *or* UN		units
ung.	*unguentum*	ointment
⊙		unit
@		at
1°		hourly
2°		2-hourly etc.
2/7		for 2 days etc.
2/52		for 2 weeks etc.
2/12		for 2 months etc.

Other abbreviations used in this book:

Abbreviation	Meaning	See chapter
B.N.F.	British National Formulary	10
B.P.	British Pharmacopoeia	10
B.S.A.	body surface area	10
I.B.W.	ideal body weight	9
SGS	standard giving set	9
v/v	volume in volume	6
w/v	weight in volume	6
w/w	weight in weight	6

Index
•••••••••••••••

Where an entry is followed by more than one page reference, the main reference is printed in **bold** type. Tables or illustrations are printed in *italic* type.

Formulae and definitions
••••••••••••••••••••••••••••••••••••••

Dosage calculations
Calculation of drug dosages   47

Drug strengths or concentrations
'1 in . . . . .' concentrations   80
mg/ml concentrations   79
Percentage concentration   74

Intravenous therapy
Calculating infusion rates
  (drops/min)   133
Calculating the length of time for I.V.
  infusions   151
Conversion of dosages to infusion
  rates   142
Conversion of infusion rates to
  drops/min   136
Conversion of ml/hour to dosages   147
Syringe drivers, setting the rate   163
  increasing the rate   164, 165

Moles and millimoles
Conversion of mg/litre to
  millimoles   119
Conversion of mg/ml to
  millimoles   119

Conversion of percentages to
  millimoles   122
Definition of moles and millimoles   119

Percent and percentages
Decimals to percentages   59
Fractions to percentages   58
Percentage of a number   59
Percentage of one number of
  another   59
Percentages to decimals   59
Percentages to fractions   59

Preparation of solutions (dilutions)
Conversion of strengths to
  percentages   104
Dilution of a stock solution of a stated
  strength   97
Preparation of soaks   104
Simple dilutions   96

Units and equivalences
Conversion of a larger unit to a
  smaller unit   37
Conversion of a smaller unit to a
  larger unit   38